Body in Balance

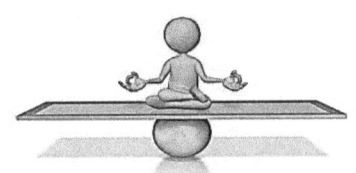

by David Dansereau, MSPT
Amazon Best Selling Author
Preventive Medicine

Copyright Notice

All rights reserved. No part of this publication may be reproduced or transmitted by any form or any means, including electronic, scanning, photocopying or recording without prior written permission. Any requests to do so must be approved by the author and owner of this work, David Dansereau, MSPT.

© 2015 PTC Physical Therapy,LLC / Smart Moves PT and David Dansereau
ISBN-13: 978-1505477092
ISBN-10: 1505477093

Table of Contents

Preface
- ABOUT THE AUTHOR
- Dedication
- Acknowledgements

Introduction
- VERY IMPORTANT - READ THIS FIRST
- Disclaimer
- Note of Results
- Getting Started is Easy

Try a New Approach
- Overcoming Barriers to Getting Started
- Deciding to Do It
- Stages of Behavior Change

Set SMART Goals

Body Composition
- How to Measure Body Fat

Other Body Biomarkers of Health

All About Metabolism
- How to Measure Your Metabolism
- How to Boost Metabolism
- Metabolic Syndrome- A Body Out of Balance

Smart Moves Fitness
- Aerobic and Strength Exercise
- Smart Movement Screen
- Smart Walk-Run Progressions
- Smart Brain Fitness

Improve your Posture Flexibility and Breathing

Smart Moves Nutrition is about Eating Clean
- Commit to Breakfast
- Our Most Vital Nutrient
- Put Smart Energy In
- Carbs
- Low Carb Debate
- Sugar Bombs
- Fats
- More on Omega 3's
- Protein
- The scoop on Paleo
- Vitamins and Minerals
- The Only Time to Fast
- Exchange your Notion of Being on a Diet
- Add Greens - Remove GMOs

Case Studies: Bodies Back in Balance

Stress Inflammation and Disease Connection
- Eat Clean: Foods that Reduce Inflammation
- How Chronic Stress Damages Your Brain
- 5 Simple Strategies to Lower Stress
- Less Caffeine
- More Sleep

References and Resources on Obesity
- Summary: Weight Loss Guidelines
- Weight Management University
- Bright Minds Kids Campaign
- More Online Resources for this Book

GMO Nation

Wrap Up-What Does this Naked Truth Mean

5 Star Customer Reviews

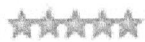

<u>5 Stars</u>- **"A Must Read for Those Ready to Eat Better"**

"David Dansereau has written an educated and informed book on the American way of eating that is clear and accessible to non-scientists. This is a must read for all those serious about their health - and their children's health. As a clinical nutritionist and physical therapist, Dansereau is well acquainted with the maladies of modern living. His well-researched evidence is quite convincing and motivating for all those who wish to change their eating for good health and longevity".-Marjorie W.

<u>5 Stars</u>- **"A practical, no-hype user manual for health and well-being"**

"Occasionally, a book comes along that has the potential to change millions of people's lives in a profound way. Body in Balance is one of these books. David Dansereau has distilled his 25 years of nutrition and physical therapy expertise into this practical, no-hype user manual for health and fitness. If you're serious about your family's health and well-being, read this book often, use the tools and resources, and put your fitness plan into action with David's guidance. You'll look better, feel great and live each day with renewed vigor and enthusiasm."-Jeff B.

<u>5 Stars</u>- **" Treat Yourself to This Great Read! "**

"I am amazed at the genuine care and compassion that David Dansereau continues to pour into his own life's mission; to educate and empower us all to live the most active, healthy, rewarding lifestyle possible. David's book

provides great explanations and insight into what educated choices we can make for ourselves and why we should! It truly is a must read! You won't be disappointed!" -Danielle Z.

<u>5 Stars</u>- **"Body in Balance...Brilliant!"**

"This book is an absolute must if you've been looking to finally get an overall balance in your HABITS. That's what it trains you to do. Find a habit, a lifestyle to follow for both healthy eating and living. The stigma of a healthy lifestyle is all in the mind, and David dives deep into this! A brilliant read for anyone struggling and needing a blueprint of healthy eating designed to help prevent any and all diseases."- Casey Z.

<u>5 Stars</u>- **"AMERICANS desperately need to Pay Attention!"**

"Americans desperately need to pay attention and read this guide! Dansereau makes it easy to understand how proper diet and the importance of daily exercise can improve over all well being. He provides sound evidence for a healthy foundation. Passionate and decisive on mind body connection. Great read for anyone who is interested in having the tools for a 2015 lifestyle adjustment."-LAD

<u>5 Stars</u>- **"David Dansereau's approach to the whole person is only part ..."**

"David Dansereau's approach to the whole person is only part of what makes him a unique practitioner. Body in Balance gives all of us access to David --a true gift for anyone who wants to understand and make sense of whole, healthy approaches to living."- Bev W.

<u>5 Stars</u>- **" love what you have put together "**

"Thank you so much David, what an inspiration, love what you have put together."- Diane W.

<u>5 Stars</u>- **"David Dansereau's expertise provides great insight into what is proven to get us off balance"**

"A book you won't want to miss in order to get your own "body in balance"! Informational and motivating, David Dansereau's expertise provide great insight into what is proven to get us off balance. This book is one of a kind as it provides the keys to optimal nutrition and points out the culprits that may be holding us back. Full of enlightening information that is to be shared with anyone and everyone you care about. What a gift! Thank you for sharing yours David! This is literally a life saver! Don't keep it a secret!"- Sue W.

Preface

The Naked Truth

The American diet couldn't be a better breeding ground if we intentionally designed it to grow cancer, heart disease and stroke as well as to fast-track diabetes. Our poor diets and the acidic environment they create for our blood encourage these illnesses and we could not have made a better experiment (our diet) if we designed it for that research purpose. But this isn't an experiment. This is your health and your vitality is slipping away every time you try to treat another symptom with yet another pill. Each of those little aches, pains, and subtle low-grade annoyances are "warning signals" that an imbalance or deficiency exists somewhere in your biochemistry, oftentimes years before it surfaces as a diagnosable condition. The first place to look for clues is your diet. Currently the standard American diet (or "SAD" as it is rightfully known by) has degenerated to the point where 62% of calories are from refined foods and about 26% come from animal products. Of that mere 10% that remains from unrefined plant food, half of that comes from white potato products which don't quite have the best nutrient density. Americans are just not eating for energy, and the numbers to follow couldn't paint a poorer picture for a Nation slipping deeper into a nutrition debt that will eventually bankrupt the US. The diet analysis mentioned is devoid of life and energy but somehow we continue to expect dead packaged foods to sustain life. They simply can't. They only add to a growing balance sheet of debt for our health in cataclysmic proportions. Those that are profiting, in addition to the pharmaceutical companies, are those selling to a "caffeine Nation" with products that aim to "fix" our extreme fatigue epidemic. The real answer begins with what you are putting on your plate.

Our growing nutrition debt concerns me, especially since illness from our forks is being adopted early on by our young bright minds.

Since the last edition of my book, the rise in the number of overweight people in the United States has become an even larger health issue as well as a growing fiscal concern. Most recent estimates show that nearly 68%, or more than two thirds of the adult population is now either overweight or obese. This is an alarming statistic in itself but it is compounded by the fact that this figure, when compared to just ten years ago, suggests that our nation has grown even 20% "fatter" in a relatively short time span. Some recent estimates suggest that of the 68% of overweight adults almost 35%, or more than one third are also considered obese! No wonder today the words obesity and epidemic are being mentioned in the same sentence as each year obesity results in over 300,000+ premature deaths.

According to the Centers for Disease Control and Prevention (CDC), the rate of type 2 diabetes has tripled in the past 40 years. The CDC also reports that in a 15 year period (1995-2010) the number of diagnosed diabetes cases rose by 50% in more than 42 states and more than 100% in 18 states. Type 2 diabetes used to be known as "adult onset" diabetes but that distinction is now being dropped because of the younger age of onset we are seeing today. Type 2 diabetes accounts for 90 to 95% of all diabetes cases in the US and with it, along with obesity, comes higher health care costs. For example:

The fiscal costs associated to this epidemic have conservatively been estimated at well over $160 BILLION !

Now here's what I find to be the most concerning part of these obesity trends. More than one-in-ten children are now becoming obese as early as the age of 2-5 years old. In total, approximately 17% of children (ages 2 to 19) are obese and 32% were either overweight or obese. While adult obesity rates have more than doubled in the past 35 years, childhood obesity rates have more than TRIPLED !

In addition to eating dead diets, perhaps the biggest cause for the growing obesity epidemic is the fact that so few people exercise. One very alarming exercise statistic published by the Centers for Disease Control and Prevention (CDC) estimates that over 80% of U.S. adults do not perform the minimum amount of exercise needed to prevent diseases, such as type II diabetes and high blood pressure. And although the benefits of exercise are well-documented, over 30 % of adults do not perform any type of exercise at all!

Is it any wonder we are sicker, fatter, and more tired than ever before. However, I remain optimistic there is a way out of this nutrition debt. The solution has nothing to do with eating more protein, eliminating carbs, or jumping on the latest Hollywood or office diet fad. In many ways, the solution to rebuilding a balanced body starts between your ears and gaining the skillpower to make change happen. Yes, there will need to be a few nutrition tweaks to cleanse your body's internal mess and reconsider what you put into your shopping cart and lift with your forks. The solution won't make you buy supplements, powders or prepackaged meals either. I can promise you'll need to swallow one pill, the "E" pill, but you won't have to flip tires, climb up ropes, or do 100 burpees with each dose!

I've found doctors don't know how to prescribe the "E" Pill correctly

By "E" Pill, I am referring to exercise. It would in fact be the most widely prescribed medicine in the world if only doctors could get it in script form for their patients! Sure, your doctor may tell you "get some exercise", but what effect does this actually have in getting you moving? If you have had a conversation like this with your doctor I guess you might consider yourself lucky. It was recently found in a national survey that less than one-third of overweight patients reported receiving advice from their doctors to increase their physical activity. At least your doctor discussed it with you, right? As far as the effect, well without a formal plan this advice has minimal effect. It has been reported that of the individuals who do receive advice, less than 10% receive help for formulating a specific activity or fitness plan, and even fewer receive follow-up support. Perhaps much of this is due to the fact that doctors and their support staffs are busy, have little knowledge about proper exercise techniques, or are currently inactive too. In fact, a recent report mentioned that in the US the average wait time to see your doctor was well over an hour, and on average, the patient had less than 30 seconds face time with their doctor to actually get their questions answered.

It is no surprise that writing a prescription for a pill solution has become the only intervention most doctors have time for in the current medical model. Mostly, it is not their fault either. The current medical practice model under third party insurance control is broken. It has most medical practitioners and the institutions they work for so bogged down in mindless paperwork and treating by codes and reimbursable practice patterns instead of by human need.

Where do you turn?

If we are not getting this vital exercise information from our doctors, where is it coming from? Well, let's be honest, unless we are told by a doctor that we have developed a certain disease or have been faced with a recent illness, most of us are concerned with our physical condition for two reasons. We care about what others see and think about us or what the mirror shows us daily. These observations might best be explained by the two most biologically driven forces in our lives that shape our behaviors-pleasure and pain.

I would see these forces or behaviors played out in my private practice daily. For example, the client that comes to me in a panic emergency state saying that he needs to lose weight and "get on a diet" because his doctor just informed him he will be facing bypass surgery unless dramatic lifestyle changes are made. The motivator in this case is the avoidance of potential pain associated with the possibility of surgery, or the feelings of pain associated with the fear of loss of income, family or both.

Although not as powerful a motivator as the avoidance of pain, I also see the other driving emotion played out very often in my practice and that is the need to change behavior in a quest to find pleasure in a better body image. While this preoccupation with external appearance may motivate some clients to achieve a healthy body, the greatest result I see in my practice is a reflection perhaps of a society of frustrated individuals with distorted perceptions of themselves who try to seek an unrealistic body shape.

Here come the hucksters again, only this time they are exercise experts!

It is exactly these two emotions that the hucksters of the infomercial marketing for fitness and weight loss products key in on. Unfortunately, it is also through these misleading advertisements and marketing channels that many consumers become misinformed. In fact, it is through these sources that most individuals get the majority of their diet and exercise "education". This advice surfaces through Madison Avenue models that determine which look is "in" each year, through the never ending array of health products, supplements, and magazines that stock the shelves of stores, and unfortunately even in the fitness industry through its amoral promise of achieving the perfect body. With all this media exposure, it's hard to convince a "normal person" to maintain a positive self-image amid a sea of perfect poster objects and "waif-like" fashion models with abhorrently low levels of body fat. No wonder so many of us have quit in disgust, or not even got motivated to try, and the record numbers of obesity today back this evidence.

The simple truth is, though impossible to shield yourself from all this nonsense, you can maintain a positive self-image by accepting what you cannot change and improving where you can. By setting realistic goals and making only personal comparisons, you'll gain both a healthy body and improved self-esteem. And although you'll hear this again, (and hopefully have heard it before) there's no quick and easy route to good health and fitness. To be healthy and strong requires a commitment to regular exercise, nourishing your body with clean nutritionally sound fuels, and adequate rest. It's not what many of us want to hear, but it is certainly the only way to restore a body to balance.

In an ideal world, everyone would interpret their own body image not through the bathroom scale or even the mirror but through their own individual measures of health and fitness. Caring about our appearance is important and can be a significant motivator. But more important is building strong muscles and bones, developing and maintaining a strong heart and brain and a flexible musculature. Formulating a balanced plan that reduces the risks of disease includes providing ourselves with nourishing foods, introducing corrective exercises and feeling relaxed and energized by getting more restorative sleep. That's what this guidebook is all about, which you'll discover.

This guidebook will review the physiology and rationale for exercise and the science behind smart nutrition, but more importantly my intention is to provide useful tweaks to get you moving in the right direction in each of these areas. I've packed this guidebook with all the latest information necessary for an individual to make lasting changes, and I've planned for its expansion and timely periodic updates which the unique companion e-book format, along with the included free webinars and resource links reinforce. Also in this new edition, I have included some of my research on genetic engineering and our food supply, and provide some evidence for why you may want to know and remove GMO foods from your plate right away. One other significant addition to this edition is my Smart Movement screen. It includes 3 simple movement patterns that you can try at home to gauge your mobility and test your balance, one of the leading causes for falls and disability as we age.

Please write me to let me know what you think of this latest update and share your success. Thank you for making a healthy purchase as well trusting me to share my knowledge and experiences with you.

Enjoy the Journey,

David P. Dansereau, MSPT

About the Author

David Dansereau is a nutritionist and licensed physical therapist. He is the president and owner of PTC Physical Therapy Consulting. He has held memberships in the American Council on Exercise, the American Dietetic Association, the International Dance and Exercise Association, the Sports and Cardiovascular Nutritionists Dietetic Practice Group, as well as the American Physical Therapy Association. He has served as Vice President for the PFO Research Foundation and volunteers as a spokesperson for Tedy's Team of the American Heart and Stroke Association.

Over more than 25 years, David has targeted his health and fitness programming to inactive individuals who are interested in beginning safe and effective exercise and nutrition programs. He had established a private practice to develop and package rehabilitation and wellness programs to teach clients how to commit to better health and physical well-being (without having to be intimidated by the typical "health club scene" and all its pressures to fit in.) Instead, David's clients are instructed one to one and learn what they might expect from their body with proper eating and therapeutic exercise. Part of this education process often involves dispelling many of the myth-conceptions of the missing "secret health ingredients" promoted by food faddists and fitness quacks.

Because of the time and attention it takes to work individually, David has developed this *Smart Moves Guidebook series* to share some of the insights on therapeutic exercise training and sensible nutrition which are the safest, most proven and effective methods available. In addition, David offers an online nutrition and exercise education course called Weight Management University, or WMU101 with an expanded interactive education and advanced coaching. David recently founded Bright Minds Kids, a health and fitness based educational initiative to introduce better nutrition and brain/body health awareness programming into schools. He is also the founder of Know-Stroke.org, a resource for stroke recovery, rehabilitation and prevention.

David has written articles for *Stroke Smart* Magazine and *Advance* for Physical Therapists. His story of stroke recovery has also been featured in the *New York Times*, on *Fox/ABC News*, as well as in *PT Products Online* Magazine.

David's Mission Statement:

"I believe there is an athlete inside us all and I believe in enabling all individuals to do the things they never thought possible. I believe education and understanding your condition are VITAL to your empowerment. I believe in treating the cause of a problem- rather than just the symptoms you might feel. And I believe that nothing should stand in the way of accomplishing **ANY goal you have**, *including your own marathon if you desire."*

Dedication

Although his hard working hands are now resting, the skills which he has passed on to me will endure. I dedicate this book in loving memory of my dad. Many times in writing this book I heard his voice reminding me to "Keep the Faith". May his spirit endure as a guiding light in my life and the lessons I learned from him be passed to my children in the stories I am able to share with them.

In loving memory of my father and coach Al Dansereau

Acknowledgements

My Sincere Thanks

First I want to thank my wife Lisa who has been right by my side and has been my hero for over 22 years. Lisa understands me like no other person in this world and was right there for me when I went through one of the most challenging periods of my life after my stroke. She has helped make this book and my online resources a reality by allowing me the time to write and rehabilitate my brain. Much of what is in this guidebook came from my own research and experimentation to heal my brain and get back in the game after my stroke. I am grateful to have found my true companion in my wife Lisa.

Thank you as well to my daughter Allison and my sons Jake and Jared who give me such pleasure and make me constantly strive to be a better person. I am so blessed to have Lisa and my children in my life.

I also want to thank you- and all the patients I have been privileged to help and work with over the years. Without you, there wouldn't be a book.

Introduction

You CAN build a better body, regardless of your age or current fitness level...

Welcome to the new updated version of Body in Balance. My goal is to show you how to boost your nutrition and fitness IQ so you'll be able to build a better body and be more fit. In this new edition, I have included new information on genetically engineered (GE) foods, food policy updates and new science, included an expanded update a my home Smart Movement screen with video links, and provided even more links to corrective exercise videos in my new SmartMovesPT home exercise platform. I've also loaded up more webinars and great nutrition documentaries to back up my research and help you keep learning. With these new resources, I'll take you through the important and necessary steps to keep you accountable and engaged and along with some new support technologies I can now offer you one-one coaching remotely to help refine the appropriate level of activity which is comfortable and effective for you. I will also help you with quick nutrition tweaks to help you build your own sensible eating plan to compliment your new fit lifestyle and along the way explain why you are likely to be misinformed when it comes to nutrition. This program will educate you on how to train your body to lose excess body fat through exercise and maintain better health regardless of your age or current fitness level.

Very Important
Read this First

Please remember, not all of the advice in this guidebook or linked to my websites from this guidebook are suitable for everyone. Because individual health and fitness levels vary considerably, you should ALWAYS consult your physician before you begin this or any weight management or exercise program.

I have provided several useful screening forms and questionnaires for assisting you with communicating with your medical expert before you get started. I would advise that you refer to these forms immediately before proceeding with taking any actions outlined in this guidebook.

Even with these assessment tools and screening forms, your physician is still your best resource for helping you decide how to best proceed with the pace of your health, fitness or rehabilitation planning.

In general, you'll find that most physicians will agree they should have to give you a prescription NOT to exercise. Someone once quoted this saying and I agree 100% with this philosophy.

"If exercise could be bottled it would be the most widely prescribed pill in the world." -Unknown

If you have completed the forms and talked about your plan with your doctor, then let's proceed.

So are you ready to look and feel better? Are you ready to have more energy?

Let's get Started!

David Dansereau

Disclaimer

This guidebook is not intended to provide medical advice on personal specific health matters, which should be provided by a qualified health care provider such as your primary care physician. The information found in this guidebook is provided solely for informational purposes and is not intended to be used for any other purpose.

Immediately discontinue any exercise which causes discomfort and consult a medical expert.

The information on this site is intended for general reference purposes only and is not intended to address any medical or health conditions. This information is not a substitute for professional medical advice or a medical exam. No health information on this guidebook should be used to diagnose, treat, cure or prevent any medical condition. The content, organization, graphics, design, compilation, magnetic translation, digital conversion and other matters related to the book are protected under applicable copyrights, trademarks and other proprietary (including but not limited to intellectual property) rights. The copying, redistribution, use or publication by you of any such matters or any part of the book, except as allowed by permission is strictly prohibited. You do not acquire ownership rights to any content, document or other materials viewed through the book. The posting of information or materials in this book does not constitute a waiver of any right in such information and materials.

Copyright 2015 / All Rights Reserved
PTC Physical Therapy Consulting
ISBN-13: 978-1505477092
ISBN-10: 1505477093

Note of Results

About Your Own Results

Not all results or case studies reflected here provide a personal guarantee of your own success. This guidebook makes no promises it can not keep. Individual results may vary and are often a result of the effort you put in.

"Nothing Happens Until Something Moves"

-Albert Einstein

This is true in physics as well as in health. In other words the laws of health are similar to the laws of physics. Just as it takes more energy to move a stationary object than a moving object, it takes a lot more time to create a successful health plan that's new, than one with a track record and a roadmap to follow. I hope you learn from the words in this book and use them to move your health forward.

Getting Started is Easy

If you are concerned that you will need to learn and do everything in this plan to be successful, then do not worry. You can begin anywhere in this guidebook or select a topic from the index and proceed at your own pace with whatever interests you.

You may even find that for now, all you have time for is a quick summary. That's O.K.! If you want to start slow, I'd suggest looking at the *Did you know...* facts at the footer of many of the pages. This may slowly get you "warmed up" and wet your appetite to the concepts in the book.

What is important is that you eventually act on the new knowledge that you have gained. You may learn from completing the exercises in this plan that you are already doing many things correctly.

Try a New Approach

If the title of my guidebook alone "_Body in Balance_" didn't alert you then I'll remind you the focus of my work is helping you acquire the "skillpower" to restore balance and achieve active changes in metabolism through smart nutrition and increased physical activity. This is the solution to sensible weight management (NOT DEPRIVATION!) which the "quick fixers" and popular diet plans may have failed to mention.

Along with some sound nutritional advice based on reality, the tools and resources found in this guide are intended help those people who have been cheated by diets succeed at lasting weight management (as well as the couch potatoes who haven't moved over the years), and inspire a few more people to throw away their bathroom scales in return for a healthier and sensible approach.

Ultimately, the goal is to provide the tools needed to build a better balanced body. In many cases mentioned already this guide may also serve as a repair manual for fixing a sluggish metabolism altered by poor nutritional habits, dead and toxic foods, or an unbalanced physical body needing a tune-up to correct faulty postures through proper therapeutic exercise education.

Regardless, we are all entitled to know the scientific facts we need to achieve or improve upon our current health. The goal of this guidebook is to provide you just that, a heads-up approach to regular exercise and smart nutrition tweaks to realign your body and improve your health and reduce your risk of some of the diseases associated with lack of activity and poor nutrition planning.

Armed with the facts and some easy -to- follow guidelines needed to achieve lasting results, it is possible to make the necessary lifestyle changes that result in a healthier body composition, improved physical fitness, self-esteem and enhanced personal appearance.

Do you Know?

What is the #1 problem people report as a barrier to adopting healthy behaviors?

Answer (or excuse?): Lack of time

"All parts of the body which have a function, if used in moderation and exercised in labors in which each is accustomed, become thereby healthy, well-developed and age more slowly, but if unused and left idle they become liable to disease, defective in growth, and age quickly."

— Hippocrates

Overcoming Barriers to Getting Started

No Time For Your own Health ?

By far the most common reason given for not practicing healthy behaviors is "There's no time!" Whether it be making time for exercise or preparing healthy meals, lack of time appears to be the most fatal common denominator. The truth, however, is that exercise is mostly a time *saver*.

Regular exercise is associated with higher levels of energy throughout the day, with increased mental clarity and focus, and with increased life span. Energy and focus will make your non-exercise time far more productive than it would be if you avoid exercise and, whatever your goals, a longer, healthier life span will help you achieve more in the long run. Add in a few good meals every day and WOW!- what a powerful punch you may be missing as a natural energy booster.

The reality is in almost every case, the excuse that "There's no time!" really means "It's not a priority!" There will be no time for exercise and proper meal planning if every other activity is more important.

Here are three <u>Action Steps</u> that use simple strategies to make sure that you have plenty of "time for your OWN health."

1. First, find ways to integrate your exercise time and meal planning with your other priorities. For example, if it is a priority to spend time with your

children, then find activities that you can do with them - like family bike rides or family meals.

2. Second, make sure that you have clearly defined goals and that you understand the importance of exercise and good nutrition. Clear goals and a commitment to a healthy lifestyle will help ensure that exercise proper nutrition stays high on your priority list.

3. Focus on the positive aspects of exercise. For example- "it's my quiet time" and "I feel great when I'm in shape" rather than focusing on the barriers to exercise like "it's so boring!", "the gym is too expensive".

The best way to adopt healthy behaviors is to keep these tips in mind. Remember, a healthy lifestyle isn't just something you do - it is something you are. Use the action steps in this guide to begin checking off your own list.

<u>Remember</u>: You can't manage what you can't measure. Take the time now to identify your goals so you have something measurable to strive for.

Deciding to Do It

What's your "Why"?

So if you have decided you are ready to do it (find your WHY) let's begin by first taking a closer look at how diet and exercise behaviors are shaped and what health professionals know about how they are changed.

I refer to this as tapping into your own "W" or finding the real **Why** behind your behavior. It is essential that you record your own goals to help understand your own individual why, or root cause, as it relates to both your accountability and motivation level- the keys to your success.

If you failed at weight loss or adopting a similar healthy behavior in the past it was probably because other things in your life were more important at the time or motivated you more than your why for changing your body and becoming healthy.

Turning W's into M's

Your M's are your motivation (not M&M's, sorry). The dictionary defines motivation as "an incentive, inducement, or motive, especially for an act." The act of changing behavior can be challenging and difficult but with the right motivation, you can attain your weight and fitness goals. Here are some tips to keep your motivation going strong, all day long.

Move
Your motivational levels are directly related to your energy levels. Physical activity releases brain chemicals, called endorphins, which enhance your sense of well being. Exercise will give you a sense of control in your life, which will ultimately enhance your sense of self-esteem and accomplishment. Keep this "feel good" chain reaction going with regular exercise.

Mind-Set
The strength of your motivation is directly related to your belief that you can succeed. "If you can think it, you can do it". If your goals are practical you will indeed be able to succeed! Hope and the power of positive thinking are the foundation of motivation. It is important to remember however that hope alone will not do it. Hope alone is not a plan. You need a plan to succeed.

Map your goals
How do you want to feel and look 3 months from now? In 6 months? One Year?
Write down your short term weight and health goals now.

Below each goal record the specific steps that must be taken in order to achieve it, such as meal planning, food shopping, healthy snacking, aerobic exercise, strength training - when, where, how often. This list will affect the way you spend your time and establish priorities. In addition, this list will help you focus on what matters most to you in your life (your w-spot) by providing a road map for you to follow to find it.

Mental picture
Motivation gives us desire. You can create the desire with the mental picture of a life full of health and fitness.

Conjure up your mental picture often and use it to get you through the day.

Membership
Stay motivated with support from my free webinars online. Membership is free for one year with the purchase of the ebook version of this guide and provides so many ways to keep you motivated. You can learn about new apps to track your progress, record your goals, access corrective exercise videos, talk with me as well as a support community in the members forum, and receive weekly newsletters.

Monitor your success
Track your weight, take your body measurements, or hang onto a pair of old jeans that used to be your size. Take a moment to look back at your success, how many positive changes you have made. Be proud of yourself!

One final word on M&M's:

Did you know? (1 M&M = 1 Football Field)
You have to walk the distance of one football field to burn off the calories you consume with one single M&M....worth it?

Stages of Behavior Change

How to interpret your motivation for exercise

In assessing your ability and interest to make a healthy lifestyle change, it is important to know that all of us generally go through a process which health professionals refer to the "Stages of Motivational Readiness for Change".

This model consists of the following stages:

Pre-contemplation -Individuals in this stage are not physically active and have not given much thought to becoming active.

Contemplation -Individuals in this stage are currently inactive but are thinking about becoming physically active.

Preparation -Individuals in this stage are physically active but not at the recommended level.

Action -Individuals in this stage are physically active at the recommended levels but typically have been doing so for only a few months.

Maintenance -Finally, individuals in this stage have typically been at the recommended level for at least 6 months.

These stages can be used as a framework to assess your own readiness for change. It is important to recognize that these are not truly linear stages, and most people make multiple attempts before they are able to achieve significant lasting change.

Where do you fit?
You purchased this book (or were given it) to read and are now doing so. If you are reading this, you are at a minimum in the contemplation stage -Correct?? Well, not so fast-keep reading!

These stages can be a little tricky because you would think that everyone would at least be in the contemplation or maybe preparation phases because they've taken some action to read about a behavior change.

But consider the following scenario: That same person, let's say his name is "Joe" who came in for a case of gout was told by his doctor that he has pre-diabetes, borderline high cholesterol and had gained 15 pounds in the last year. The physician highly recommended Joe start adopting a more active lifestyle to help manage and hopefully prevent going on medications for these conditions. Joe explains that he doesn't enjoy exercise and has a job that involves many late evenings, a lot of travel, and too much "on the go" eating when healthy food options aren't always available. In fact, the only reason why Joe agreed to meet with his doctor is because he promised his spouse he would. And maybe it was even his spouse who bought Joe my book!

What stage of change do you think Joe is in?

If you chose precontemplation, you're correct. Someone who is in precontemplation does not see the value in exercise, and perceives more cons than pros in adopting a healthier lifestyle. As a physical therapist, when I encounter someone in the precontemplation stage like Joe, I don't push too hard into exercise recommendations because his (or her) mind is closed to it. Instead, I would use my time during Joe's therapy to make inactivity relevant by educating him or her on all of the risks associated with inactivity and how activity can have a positive impact (reduce joint pain, decrease stress,etc.) so hopefully Joe will start to consider being physically active, or at least think about completing a few of his PT home exercises!

Bottom Line: It takes time and it takes practice to master these skills, so it is important to understand the concept of lapses and relapses. I want to assure you that straying from your diet and exercise plan is not a failure or a reason to give up. Either is taking a break from my book for a bit, as long as you learn a few new skills and eventually put them into action! When you pick up where you left off, I will be here to help you get back on track:) This is one of the main reasons why I structured this book loosely in categories, I want you to be able to flip through it and "digest" small bits of good information to help get your Body in Balance.

What to do if you are in the precontemplation stage?

Is this you? You are not even considering changing. You may be "in denial" about your health problem or lack of initiative, or not consider it serious. You may have tried unsuccessfully to change so many times that you have given up.
What you can do! Educate yourself on risks versus benefits and positive outcomes related to change.

What to do if you are in the contemplation stage?

Is this you? You are ambivalent about changing. But... you find yourself weighing the benefits versus costs or barriers (e.g., time, expense, bother, fear) of change.
What you can do! Identify barriers and misconceptions- Address concerns and identify support systems.

What to do if you are in the preparation stage?

Is this you? You are prepared to experiment with small changes.
What you can do! It is time to develop realistic goals and timeline for change. Prepare by finding a support team/system for positive reinforcement and begin to make them part of your plan.

What to do if you are in the preparation stage?

Is this you? You are taking definitive action to change behavior.
What you can do! Stick with resources and the people that provide positive reinforcement.

What to do if you are in the Maintenance stage?

Is this you? You have been striving to maintain the new behavior over the long term, let's say approximately 6 months or more.
What you can do!
Congratulations! Continue to stick with resources and people that provide positive reinforcement. Build your team, take on new challenges by setting new and perhaps more internally rewarding goals.

Set SMART Goals

How to do it SMART!

To reach your goals you have to have your "why" identified first to get clear on what you want to achieve. To get more specific you should use the acronym, and the lead word in the title of this book, 'SMART'. To check if your goals are smart, follow this guide:

Specific
The reason for being specific is to uncover your true "why", or ultimate goal as well as the reasons behind it. During a difficult time in your life you may have gained weight. A goal to lose 10 pounds, for example, is specific, but let's investigate *why* losing 10 pounds is the right goal to begin with. If you had more energy from being lighter and could move your extremities easier to exercise them more, would that be more appealing than what the scale reads? Perhaps it is not so much the number (10 pounds) but the increased energy, decreased pain and good feeling that would come from the process in attempting to lose the weight. So, your *why* for weight loss may really be to make it easier to move your body to exercise for 15 more minutes daily. You may find that the goal itself is now completely different from what it started out to be.

Measurable
If your goal is to "walk faster", it will be difficult to assess when you have actually reached your goal unless you set measurable benchmarks to provide you with specific

feedback (daily, weekly or monthly) on your
progress. Create a log or movie of your walking progress
and record the number of minutes walked each day, days
walked per week, as well as distance traveled and any
help needed. Record your mood and energy level to help
remind you how you felt when you reached a new walking
level or hit a plateau. If you cannot measure a goal, you
do not know what is working and cannot adjust what you
are doing.

Action-Oriented
How are you going to reach your goal? Planning action
steps will provide the blueprint to the end goal. To "walk
faster", what specific walking workout is best for
you? How often? Which strength and flexibility exercises
should be performed for which muscles? What foods
would provide the best energy for your workouts? The
action steps provide the answers to your unique
questions and will lead you toward your ultimate
goal. Don't overlook the process of recording action
steps. Develop 5 to 8 small action steps to help lead you
in the right direction towards your ultimate goal.

Realistic
Keep your goals within the realm of possibility and make
them relevant, or you will get discouraged. Let's go back
to the weight loss goal again of losing 10 pounds.   If you
give yourself one week to lose the weight it is not only
unrealistic but could be potentially dangerous. Believe
you can achieve but be flexible in the process. If you are
attempting to attain a rehabilitation goal in a short time
frame, you will only increase the level of stress and
possibly lose sight of why you started the goal process.

Time Frame
Set a time frame for your goal. Write a goal down on
paper and put it on your calendar and also in an

additional visible location where you can see it daily. Post it to your refrigerator, computer screen or bathroom mirror, or record this goal date in your goal movie and play it often. You need to be reminded daily of your commitments and actions. Without a time frame, your goal will only be a wish. It is certainly OK to keep the faith and wish, but record a timeline to help you keep the focus too. Don't just wish for it, live for it! Having Hope is a Good Quality to stay positive, but it is a mindset and not a plan. To achieve any goal and give the best odds at lasting change requires a plan.

SMART GOAL SETTING TIPS:

1. Find a proven path from an authentic teacher, coach or person you look up to who has gotten the results you desire and can prove it and/or teach it to you. Also may be effective to hire a coach or teacher if you need help to make you focus and keep you accountable.*
2. Create a movie dedicated to your SMART Goals. Here's why:
    - Keeps track of success and failure by recording progress
    - Helps you view before /after results
    - Helps motivate and increase adherence to goals
    - Provides valuable record to show your doctors, therapists, and yes perhaps even your health insurance provider, as they now are becoming more willing to actually pay for wellness!

Reason for the movie: Subconscious mind/your emotional side think in pictures. Turn your goal into a success movie to help motivate you!

Example:
Combine multiple goals into one compelling, continuous internal movie.
Describe your goal and put yourself "INSIDE" the movie and then practice adding more sensory elements. What did you hear? What did you smell?

To see a sample of this plan in action here's a link to my SMART goal setting outline I used following my stroke to prepare to run the Boston Marathon. You can watch the webinar replay at http://www.know-stroke.org

*More on the Power of Accountability

Just imagine what would happen if I were to follow you with a camera crew 24 hours a day 7 days a week for the first 100 days of 2015 while you went for your goals?

I bet 3 things would happen…

1) You would START doing the things you say you need to do.

2) You would STOP doing the things you know you shouldn't be doing.

3) You would MAKE monumental performance gains and have the best year of your life.

How this possible? Through the power of accountability!

Accountability serves to protect your character, as well as your credibility, and more importantly, it helps you to accomplish all of your goals.

Did you know?
THE #1 thing that stops people from accomplishing their goals is their lack of accountability so make plans now using some of these strategies provided here to hold yourself accountable!

Body Composition

What is it you really want to lose?

Excess Body Fat! -Not lean muscle.

We all have it in our bodies. Even the leanest athletes.

We need some fat for optimal health. We all have some degree of "fatness". One's degree of fat does not necessarily imply obesity. Consequently, there are many people that are overfat, however and they may still be at "normal weight" on the scales. Losing excess fat should be the focus rather than a misleading concentration of the total weight on the scale.

What Does Your Weight Tell You

Individuals trying to lose fat often make the mistake of relying solely on the scale as a barometer of their success with weight loss. In reality, this method tells the person nothing about what they are losing. Is it fat, water, or muscle?

Don't put too much weight on the scale

If you weigh yourself at least once a day, you need to know that you're putting too **much weight or emphasis on your scale!**

Many people weigh themselves constantly in order to monitor their rate of fat loss. But if you are one of these people, you should be aware that there are factors other than body fat that influence the number that appears each time you step on the scale.

Consider these facts:

Water Weight:
The human body is comprised of approximately 60% water. So naturally, the amount of water floating around your system will have an impact on your weight. This doesn't mean you should cut down on your water intake, however. Believe it or not, the less water you take in, the more likely it is for your body to hold onto its water stores, causing you to become bloated. The way to counteract this is to actually increase your water intake. Six to eight 8-ounce glasses a day of water should be sufficient, but if you are very active, increase your water consumption to ten glasses daily.

Another reason why your body might want to hold onto water is if you consume a lot of salt. Sodium (a major component of table salt) attracts water, so the more sodium you take it, the more fluids you'll retain. The Daily Value for sodium is only 2400mg. Since a mere teaspoon of salt contains about 2000mg of sodium, you can see how easy it is to go beyond the recommended limit.

In my private practice this is one of the first key dietary modifications I suggest when working with a new patient- <u>key in on identifying and reducing sodium intake.</u> Remember, prepackaged ready-made meals and snacks are generally loaded with sodium to increase product shelf life as well as attack your taste buds so you reach for more. Once you begin eating clean however, and eliminating these dead foods, then modifying sodium intake becomes a non-issue as whole food replacements are generally low in sodium naturally.

Yes, it's true, ladies. Women do suffer from pre-menstrual water retention. Again, the best way to minimize water weight gain is to drink more, not less, water and to reduce your intake of high sodium foods.

Food Intake:
We seem to forget that food and beverages not only contain calories, but they contain mass as well. So, if you are weighing yourself after you eat a meal, don't be surprised if the scale gives a false reading of a bit more than you actually weigh. Weight yourself prior to eating.

Lean Body Mass:
If your goal is to lose weight and you recently started a strength-training program, don't be alarmed if the number on the scale refuses to budge or even (gasp!) goes up a bit. When you strength train, fluid accumulates within the muscles as part of their repair and rebuilding process, adding to their mass. Also, muscle weighs more than fat. So, even if the scale tells you that you haven't lost weight per say, there's a good chance that you have lost some fat. The best indicator of true fat loss, without having your body fat tested by a professional, is how your clothes fit you. If they feel a bit looser, you'll know you're making progress.

Remember that it takes 3,500 calories above what you already eat in order to gain just one pound of fat.

It is highly unlikely that you'll gain a pound of fat overnight!!

The best thing you can do to monitor your true weight loss (and to prevent getting upset by the expected fluctuations) is to step on that scale only once a week, not every day.

The Function of Body Fat

About half of the body's fat is found just under the skin. The other areas in the body that contain fat stores are around the major bodily organs where fat serves as protection. Also some fat is found interlaced between muscle fibers in the body, with higher quantities of fat found in muscles with low levels of activity. The fat in our bodies does have a necessary role. Fat acts as a storage reserve for when food is unavailable for extended periods of time.

As mentioned fat also insulates and protects us from cold temperatures and protects or pads our vital organs. Fat in the body helps to store the fat soluble vitamins, A,D,E and K. Controlling fat does not imply depleting the body's fat reserves so that these functions become impaired. It should imply monitoring dietary fats and keeping body fat regulated with a consistent exercise program.

The Excess Body Fat / Pain Connection

Being overweight and having excess bodyfat can certainly lead to painful joints or other problems as arthritis or injuries to the spine. There are two critical reasons why this happens.

1) Fatty tissue is an endocrine (hormone-producing) organ, just like other organs in the body. Studies show that patients who are overweight produce high levels of

cytokines, C-reactive protein and other pro-inflammatory chemical-substances that promote joint and tissue damage and increase pain.

2) In addition to fat causing these changes inside the joint, the load outside the joints of the lower extremities by the excess weight take a physical toll on soft tissues forced to try to maintain support for an overstressed skeletal system.

Did you know? For every extra pound of excess body fat a person carries around it is estimated that the joints of the lower body get that weight multiplied by a factor of 3-4 pounds. For example, a woman carrying an extra 50 pounds of excess body fat over her ideal weight/frame size can actually be placing an additional 200 pounds of pressure on her hips, knee and ankle joints all day long! It has always been my position, that as a physical therapist it is my job to let patients know these simple truths. Excess body fat matters, and trying to ignore it and treat around this truth makes no sense. If you are in need of therapy and healing for pain or for an overuse injury, you should look at your nutrition first as part of a balanced solution to recovery.

Let's look at the good news

Losing as little as 10-20 pounds of excess body fat can significantly reduce inflammation, pain and stiffness- regardless of the underlying cause of the discomfort. Clients that learned this in my clinic and combined weight loss with a diet that includes anti-inflammatory foods (and excludes pro-inflammatory ones) realized pain could reduce as much as 90%. Many were able to drop their reliance on ibuprofin and similar pain killers and avoid the gastrointestinal upset and other side effects, simply by choosing cleaner foods. I've included a chapter on the foods to fight stress and inflammation in this book.

Did you know?

According to a recent Consumer Reports (sept 2014) Americans are in pain in epidemic numbers and are reaching for more potent and deadly painkilers.

Prescriptions for pain meds have climbed 300 percent in the past decade, and Vicoden and other drugs containing the narcotic hydrocodone are now the most commonly prescribed medications in the US. Every day, 46 people in the US die from legal pain pills.

How to Measure Body Fat

Body Composition

A variety of methods to assess body "fatness" exist including underwater weighing, skinfold measurements, or using various electronic assessment techniques such as bioelectrical impedance or various ultrasound technologies. All of these tests help to gauge the fat vs. the lean tissue composition of the body.

Generally, the hydrostatic weighing method is still considered the "gold standard" for assessing the percentage of bodyfat, but the cost of this test is often prohibitive. Many new technologies and imaging devices are coming available to assess bodyfat but at the time of this publishing they are still remain too costly to enter into our discussion here.

Just as the costs involved with having body composition measured vary dramatically with each of these methods so do the results when comparing between methods. It is generally best to use one method and stick with it. The most affordable and consistent way to assess body "fatness" which I like to use in my professional practice is the skinfold caliper method.

I remember one of the first "big" investments I made when I started my private practice over 25 years ago were my skinfold calipers. I spent over $400 on these calipers and today with the advances in technology the calipers are available with the same accuracy for a cost under $40! At this price it makes home monitoring very affordable and actually quite simple to master. I've provided guidelines for you to use at the end of this chapter if you desire to monitor your own body fat at home. Alternatively, you could check at your local health club or with a health professional to see if they offer this service.

For more information on the calipers I would advise for home use along with the best price I've found on the web, go to the special web link I've set up in the resources pages.

What's in a number?

Body composition assessment (body fat assessment) can be difficult to discuss fairly because it is so intimately tied with our body perception and even our sense of self-worth. However, it is an important subject because body fat results are strongly predictive of your risk coronary heart disease, several types of cancer, stroke, diabetes, osteoarthritis, high blood cholesterol, and high blood pressure and even your metabolic rate as discussed in the chapter on your metabolism.

From an athletic standpoint, body fat levels are also closely correlated with athletic performance.

To understand your results, keep in mind that scientists typically divide body weight into fat weight and fat-free weight. The fat-free weight is primarily muscle, bone, and water.

The preferred measure of body composition is the ratio of fat weight to overall weight. For example, body fat composition results are likely to be expressed as a percentage (refer to the example which follows). This is the percentage of fat weight relative to overall body weight. This percentage gives a sense of the distribution in the body between muscle, bone and water or what together are referred to as fat-free mass versus the remainder of the body weight which is fat, also referred to as adipose tissue.

As mentioned briefly earlier, some body fat is essential for healthy living. Energy production and neurological systems, in particular, will not operate properly without some lipids (fats) in the diet and on the body.

However, the problem is that many people simply have far more body fat than is needed or appropriate for healthy living. In a clinical setting, the terms "slightly over fat", "fat" and "obese" are used to describe degrees of this excess fat accumulation.

Body Fat Rating	Men	Women
Lean (Athletes)	<8%	<13%
Optimal (Ideal Fitness)	8-15%	13-23%
Slightly Over fat	16-20%	24-27%
Fat	21-24%	28-32%
Obese	>25%	>33%

If you have a recent body fat measurement and would like to know how to interpret the results, I have provided some general population reference norms for body fat here. While our standards (or "norms") for fat are typically higher for people as they age (especially into their 40s and 50s), the following table represents a reasonable consensus view for the classification of fat levels for adults.

As a side note, many male endurance athletes fall under 8 percent bodyfat, while the threshold for females is 12 percent.

In general, body fat values under 5 percent for men and 10 percent for women are considered dangerous and unhealthy because the body has a level of essential fat needed for normal body functions which differs between sexes.

In reviewing this chart, it is essential that you distinguish between issues of body image versus issues of health. It is quite common for both men and women to be within the optimal body fat range and yet still be unhappy with their body image. However, it is also true that people may be perfectly healthy even into the "Slightly Over fat" range if they are otherwise active and eat well.

Similarly, some people discover that their body fat level is quite high even though their overall weight is quite low and, from external appearances, they are quite slim. This occurs when both activity level and food consumption are so low that lean body weight falls to a very low level.

Since health outcomes are predicted by the ratio of body fat and not the quantity of body fat, appearance alone is often not the best indicator of health risk.

Summary of key points to measure your body fat accurately

- Take all measurements on the dominant side of your body

- Carefully identify and recall your measuring site for accuracy

- Take the measurement when skin is dry and lotion-free

- Do not measure immediately after exercise due to shifts in body fluid

Sites for men: Skinfolds are taken on the chest, abdomen, and thigh.

Sites for women: Skinfolds are taken on the back of the upper arm, abdomen, and thigh.

I suggest investing in a Slimguide skinfold caliper if you'd like to measure your bodyfat regularly at home. They are inexpensive and reliable when compared to the professional investment I made for my practice. See the resources page as well as a link to a video for measuring body fat.

Other Body Biomarkers of Health

Could an "Ideal" Weight on the Scale Be Misleading?

(See the case study at the end of this chapter for a practical example and the answer!)

Height – Weight Tables

Years ago height-weight tables were popularly used to provide recommended weight ranges for a certain height. Many of these old tables are referenced from insurance companies back in the 1950's and 60's, yet some medical professionals still refer to them. Most medical professionals know better and understand that the body weight displayed from a scale as an indicator of over/underweight is sometimes misleading. It is due to the fact that body composition is different from each individual's unique characteristics including frame size, muscle construction, fluid retention and other factors which are all variable. Therefore, it is a better approach to determine your ideal weight by making use of your individual body fat percentage in relation to the body composition rating scale I provided for you.

Body Mass Index

Much like the height- weight tables, a related measure called the Body Mass Index (BMI) still plays a role in health screening. BMI attempts to show a relationship between height and weight and provide a marker to assess obesity. However, it is important to note that both BMI and height-weight tables provide only a very rough estimate of one's ideal or healthy body weight.

For example, athletic individuals with large amounts of fat-free weight (muscle) are usually defined as "overweight" when using these methods despite having low amounts of body fat and being quite healthy.

At the same time, those with small amounts of muscle and bone can often be designated as "underweight" when in actuality they may be carrying too much body fat.

For these reasons, I do not suggest using these references when a true body fat measure is available.

Current BMI Guidelines

Here are the current BMI Guidelines according to the American College of Cardiology (ACC)/American Heart Association (AHA)/The Obesity Society (TOS) 2113

Guidelines on the Management of Overweight and Obesity in Adults.

"Providers are recommended to measure height and weight and calculate BMI at annual visits or more frequently to identify patients who need to lose weight. Use of current cut points for overweight (BMI >25.0-29.9 kg/m2) and obesity (BMI ≥30 kg/m2) should be continued to identify adults who may be at increased risk for CVD (cardiovascular disease). A cut point for obesity (BMI ≥30 kg/m2) should be used to identify adults at increased risk for all-cause mortality. Patients who are overweight or obese should be counseled that their BMI level places them at increased risk for CVD, type 2 diabetes, and all-cause mortality. " I have provided more details from this report in the summary and resources section at the end of this book on weight loss guidelines.

Waist-Hip Ratio and Waist Circumference

More recently, researchers have created other measures such as the Waist-Hip Ratio and the Waist Circumference measures so that they can capture information about where excess fat is deposited. This is in response to research showing that health risks are most common in individuals whose excess fat is deposited in abdominal areas rather than the hip and thigh areas.

In other words, health risks are greater for those who have much of their body fat in the upper body, especially the trunk and abdominal areas. This is called android obesity (or apple-shaped) in comparison to gynoid obesity (or pear-shaped, characterized by deposition of fat in the hips and thighs).

The ratio of waist and hip circumferences (WHR) is a simple and convenient method of determining the type of obesity present. The risk of disease increases strongly when the WHR of men rises above 0.9, and of women, above 0.8.

Current Waist Circumference Guidelines

Guidelines for Waist Circumference according to the American College of Cardiology (ACC)/American Heart Association (AHA)/The Obesity Society (TOS) 2113 Guidelines on the Management of Overweight and Obesity in Adults:

"Waist circumference should be measured at annual visits or more frequently in overweight and obese adults. Cut points for increased waist circumference defined by the National Institutes of Health or World Health Organization (**>35 inches or 88 cm for women and >40 inches or 102 cm for men**) can be used. Patients who have an increased waist circumference should be counseled that their BMI level places them at increased risk for CVD, type 2 diabetes, and all-cause mortality."

Other important easy "DIY" (do it yourself) biomarkers of your health:

- Blood Pressure (exercise and resting)
- Heart Rate (exercise and resting)

There are great apps and online tools to help you track these biomarkers as well as help you monitor other important blood and lipid markers that can be helpful measurements to keep in your health checkbook. I've included links in the resource section.

CASE STUDY:

To answer the question I asked at the beginning of this chapter.

"Yes", an ideal weight on the scale could be misleading. In summary, here's why:

<u>The Scale Alone Can't Reveal if You're Replacing Fat with Metabolism Revving Muscle.</u>

By monitoring the changes of your lean body weight, you will be able to tell whether or not you are replacing fat with muscle. Lean body weight can be found by subtracting your body weight with your body fat weight. Your body fat weight is calculated by multiplying your weight with your body fat percentage.

Here's an example:

Susan's current weight is 180 pounds. She recently had her body fat measured at 25%.

Based upon her current weight her body composition distribution can be calculated as follows:

180 pounds (current weight) x .25 (25% body fat)=45 pounds of body fat

180 pounds (current weight) − 45 pounds of fat = 135 pounds of fat free mass (FFM) or lean body weight (LBW)

In assessing Susan's weight according to the Body Fat Rating Chart she would be rated as currently "slightly over fat" for her current weight.

Action Step

<u>Try setting a target body fat goal instead of a weight loss goal on the scale</u>

Let's take Susan in the example above. If I were working with her I would suggest a possible short term goal of initially losing 4% bodyfat to improve her rating on the body fat chart to that of "Optimal". If Susan's goal for a target body fat to get to the "Optimal" zone is 21% (and ideally she wants to preserve lean muscle and lose the excess fat), I'll perform a calculation to show what her projected new body weight would be at her new body composition. In Susan's example her new projected body weight would be approximately 171 pounds.

If you have completed your own body composition assessment at home and would like to have me assist you with setting up a realistic target body composition goal, I offer a private coaching/consulting service. Please contact me with your information and we can set up an appointment in person, online or via chat. See the resources link for more information.

All About Metabolism

One of the most vital components to good health

What is Metabolism?

Metabolism is the process by which your body uses calories to support its functions and fuel daily activity. Metabolic rate refers to how slow or fast this process of "burning" calories from food occurs. Resting metabolic rate (RMR) is the number of calories the body requires just to maintain basic body functions such as breathing, circulation and temperature regulation. Your RMR typically represents 60 to 75 percent of your total metabolic output on a daily basis. Considering this estimate it makes sense to target this area to try to improve upon if your goal is to lose body fat.

The other process that elevates your metabolism happens when your body digests food. This process is known as thermogenesis, or the "thermic effect of food", and it can contribute up to 15 percent to your total daily energy expenditure. Up to another 20 percent of your total daily energy expenditure can be accounted for by the lifestyle you lead or the level of activity you get from your occupation or formal exercise program.

Can RMR be altered?

Yes it certainly can, but to answer this question correctly we should take a closer look at some of the realities of how RMR factors in to the weight loss puzzle.

Reality and Recommendations

The average American man and woman add around one pound of body weight every year during middle age. This condition is often called "creeping obesity" because over the years the weight mysteriously sneaks up on you. Right?

Not really.

What happens to your body actually has more to do with your activity level, your diet, and your metabolism. Many people are aware of the weight gain, but few understand the cause or the real solution to the problem. Let's begin by looking at the reality of weight gain for most adults. Here's some evidence to the reality of the problem before looking at the recommendations:

Reality #1: Most adults do not exercise regularly

According to the U.S. Public Health Service Centers for Disease Control, close to <u>85 percent</u> of the American public does not get enough exercise to receive any significant therapeutic fitness benefit. Remember that valuable E-Pill I mentioned earlier?

Even when adults work in jobs they consider physically demanding, the fact is most occupations cannot provide adequate continuous fitness benefit. On the contrary, low fitness levels make every day work duties appear more demanding than they should be.

In addition, the majority of adults make the transition from a more active childhood lifestyle to a usually sedentary adult work and leisure time lifestyle. The evidence shows a sedentary behavior in adulthood begins a cycle that leads to far greater problems trying to control weight gain as you age.

Reality #2: Most adults gradually lose muscle tissue as they age

Evidence from some classic studies conducted in the 90's by Dr. Bill Evans and his work with biometrics as well as data collected by other researchers indicate that non-exercising adults lose about 5 to 6 pounds of muscle every decade of life. This age associated loss of lean muscle mass is known as sarcopenia. One of my research projects as a physical therapy grad student was to look at sarcopenia and some of Evans work. The studies Evans conducted on the elderly population were fascinating. He was able to successfully and safely introduce strength training in a population that was once considered "too old" to exercise, especially with weights. Evans proved dramatic changes could be made in physical mobility in individuals as old as 90+ years, and even documented significant gains in strength and muscle gains as well.

Muscle that is not used or that does not obtain adequate regular resistance exercise gradually gets smaller and weaker. This not only adversely influences our physical ability and functional capacity, its loss also is believed to cause a decrease in our resting metabolic rate. So perhaps then "creeping obesity" can be averted by swallowing the E-pill!

Reality #3: Most adults experience a decrease in resting metabolism.

Most of the calories our bodies expend during each day occur at rest, a lower resting metabolism means simply less energy is used throughout the day... times day after day. Remember it is estimated that 75% of the total calories we use each day are due to our RMR and up to 5% of this resting rate is "lost" every decade contributing to a lower "resting" metabolism.

Reality #4: Many adults still believe in following low calorie diets

We thought that for years the apparent solution to weight gain was simply to diet. Billions of dollars are still spent on diet programs today, even though most of the money spent is simply wasted.

Unfortunately, many diet programs (even many of the popular franchises) are still using low-calorie diets and giving little or no formal instruction for developing a comprehensive exercise program that delivers lasting results in all the components of fitness.

Reality #5: Diet programs produce temporary results and make weight gain problems only worse

Dropout rates are high and success rates are low for diets. But if that is not enough, research has discovered that dieting alone will produce <u>both</u> fat loss and <u>loss of lean tissue or muscle</u>. In fact, the proportion of fat weight to muscle weight lost can be equal on very low calorie diets.

If the basic cause of weight gain is low muscle mass, then sacrificing more muscle to a low calorie diet is clearly troublesome. This practice only lowers metabolism and when the diet can no longer be tolerated and must stop, the lost weight is regained. Only, this time the weight regained is mostly fat, and the resulting body composition and appearance is worse than before dieting.

And for the dieter that tries to hang on and continue to try to push through this cycle they often make the mistake of lowering calories even further therefore slowing metabolism even more !

Start to <u>think about</u> incorporating these recommendations:

Recommendation #1: Begin an exercise program first and include an eating plan that fuels your activity

Most studies on weight management show that a healthy diet plus exercise can decrease fat weight while increasing muscle weight. It is advisable to include regular aerobic exercise AND strength training in any weight loss program.

Recommendation #2: Strength train to promote muscle gain

A balanced exercise program which includes some form of resistance exercise should be part of your smart fitness plan. The average American adult has too much fat and too little muscle, and strength training, smart moves circuit workouts or similar muscle toning exercises are the best way to increase muscle and help speed up a sluggish metabolism.

Weight training is the only exercise that has been proven to elevate RMR for extended periods of time. Several strength training studies have shown that working out with weights elevates your "burn rate" for up to 15 hours. Compare this study to similar ones completed for aerobic exercise and you'll discover that for most cardiovascular activities lasting under 60 minutes, the "afterburn" you get from this mode of exercise only lasts for up to one hour and then your RMR returns to normal.

Recommendation #3: Learn how to distinguish fact from fiction

One of the biggest challenges we all face is getting the facts we need to know for better health. Getting rid of the myths and fads that seem to be everywhere is of great importance to making the smart moves that are actually necessary in order to pay healthy dividends.

We all want a program that takes the least time, gives the best results, and doesn't miss anything crucial. And don't be fooled, the folks that market the diet infomercials and fitness products know all too well how to push your "pain and pleasure" buttons. Unfortunately, many popular quack diets and fitness fads promise just what the consumer wants but actually waste time, money and potentially jeopardize health in the process.

David Dansereau

How to Measure Your Metabolism

Metabolism Matters: Know How Many Calories You Burn

The essential fact of weight management is that you will lose weight if you burn more calories than you eat and will gain weight if you eat more than you consume. While popular diets differ in their distribution of macronutrients (fats, carbohydrates and protein), all of these diets ultimately require a caloric deficit for weight loss.

The problem with all commercial diets is that they offer no way to calculate the calories you are burning so that you can accurately and safely select an appropriate caloric intake. Instead you are left guessing in a world where no two days of eating and activity are the same and where adjustments must be made as your body composition changes. As I mentioned in the introduction, the major mistake all commercial weight loss programs make is they place the emphasis on weight on the scale instead of focusing on achieving a healthy body composition.

Establish Realistic Goals:

I've provided 2 methods to help you define your goals. Use the Action Steps Log found in the resources link to this guide or register for my PTCMAP online activity and meal planner. In contrast to the "one calorie level fits all mentality" of the commercial weight loss centers, my online meal planning tool uses the same assessment techniques I use in my private practice to accurately measure individual caloric needs. The easy setup area of my members site includes the correct formulas to estimate your resting metabolic rate (RMR) from lean muscle mass, not just from total weight on the scale. Since my online meal planner includes all the lean muscle mass and RMR formulas built in to the program and figures it out instantly for you, it has the flexibility to be used as a self-help program or can be incorporated in with one of my executive nutrition coaching services over the web.

About metabolism measurement:

With today's technology, an expert analysis of you caloric expenditure budget or RMR can be completed in a health professionals office in 7-10 minutes through a technology called indirect calorimetry. In my private practice I use a device called the Bodygem handheld analyzer. There are now several companies that offer similar technologies to measure RMR. Once your resting metabolic rate is determined with this measurement, you'll have a safe and accurate starting point for gaining or preserving muscle and losing fat that is individually calculated for your body's needs. This unique number is sometimes referred to as knowing your metabolic fingerprint. Just like knowing your blood pressure numbers are essential to gauging the health of your heart and circulatory system, your metabolic fingerprint is a vital number essential to your weight management success.

SMART MOVE:

Measure your burn rate or resting metabolic rate.

How does metabolism measurement work?

Due to recent advances in microprocessor technology, measuring metabolism is now done quickly, accurately and easily. A portable handheld device like the Bodygem measures oxygen consumption to determine the body's metabolism while at rest and during exercise. This allows individuals monitoring their health and diet to accurately assess their caloric needs, providing better data than is possible with outdated prediction estimates.

Measuring resting metabolic rate was previously possible only in large, expensive devices found in hospitals and research clinics; now the portable and affordable measurement technologies available bring this function to the individual through the use of revolutionary oxygen and flow sensor technology. Expect to pay between $65-$150 per measurement depending on the amount of nutrition counseling provided along with your RMR result.

One way to calculate your RMR to get a quick calorie burning estimate is to use this formula:

RMR=

665+(4.36 x weight)+(4.32 x Height in inches)-4.7x age)

Note: This method does not account for all your body variables, like metabolically active lean muscle which burns oxygen / more calories at rest. When able to, use your lean muscle mass as determined from your body fat measurement and use the tool in my PTC MAP system or have your RMR measured by indirect calorimetry for best result.

How to Boost Metabolism

How to Make the Energy Balance Equation Work for You

Most commercial weight loss programs ultimately fail because they do not consider the burn side of the Energy Balance Equation

Until recently, there has not been an easy or economical way to measure metabolism or your burn rate also referred to as RMR (resting metabolic rate). People have relied on predictive equations which are inaccurate for many, particularly those on both ends of the energy balance equation. For example those who participate in strength training exercise programs (high end), or those individuals that have dieted on and off for most of their lives (low end) and have followed the typical "Yo-Yo" effect of cycling weight loss with repeated weight gain, are subject to the greatest margin of error if using prediction equations.

I provided you with a common predictive (RMR) equation if you would like to get a very general idea of your resting metabolic rate in the previous section.

Keep in mind, many apps and online calculators can also be helpful but be mindful that these estimates can be off as much as by 500 calories per day according to recent studies especially if you have a long history of "Yo-Yo" effect dieting.

The Reason Most Predictive Equations Don't Get "You":

Lean muscle burns significantly more calories than fat mass and predictive equations can't account for changes in metabolism due to improvements in overall body composition. These predictive equations therefore become quite inaccurate and too low for people on the high end of the energy balance scale, and unfortunately too high for those individuals on the low end of the scale. As you may have heard, the fatal flaw of most low calorie diets is that you end up sacrificing lean muscle. Therefore, during the next round of dieting you have actually negatively affected your body composition (lost lean and gained fat) so your dieting efforts literally ruin you with an even lower RMR due to loss of energy revving muscle.

Oxygen: The Universal Fuel of Metabolism

Our bodies use oxygen to metabolize food. So, measuring how much oxygen your body consumes tells you exactly how many calories your body burns at rest each day.

Everyone's metabolism or burn rate is unique to them- a one size fits all approach to weight loss and fitness does not work for most individuals. Take a recent study on "Predictive vs Measured RMR" as an example below:

In the study subjects of the same height, weight, age and gender were predicted to have had the same burn rate (RMR) when using the old predictive equation. When this group of women actually had their RMR measured, however, their real burn rates were dramatically different. When the Predicted vs. the Actual numbers were compared there was a significant difference, ranging from 100-500 calories on average. This helps to explain why you can follow the same exercise routine and eat the same foods as your friend, but have dramatically different results.

This is also why trying to figure out a weight loss plan based on using powders, potions, diets in a can, weight loss cookies, as well as points and prepackaged meals based upon outdated "Ideal" height/weight charts will not work in the long run to produce lasting change.

What else doesn't work?

- Avoid all over the counter supplements touted to boost your metabolism. You simply can't buy a pill solution to your sluggish metabolism.

- Avoid packaged, processed foods or weight loss solutions that require you to purchase their own brand of foods in a box. When you break down the nutrition in these foods you'll see they fall short for healthy eating.* The sulfites, sodium, nitrites, GMOs and trans fats guarantee a long shelf life, but do nothing to improve yours!

- Guessing!

What works?

Improving your metabolism or at least doing your best to maintain a high burn rate as you age. Preserving your RMR is <u>THE BEST</u> long term predictor of weight management success. Balancing diet with exercise, both cardiovascular and resistance training, is the most effective way to reach your weight management goals.

Consistent resistance training at the correct intensity increases your lean muscle mass and increases your resting metabolic rate.

Cardiovascular training burns extra calories and contributes to your total daily calorie expenditure. Get plenty of rest, build in time in your day for fun activities, and drink plenty of pure water. Educate yourself and your family about the benefits of healthy eating and using more whole food nutrition. While supplements may be able to help with some of the nutrients you need they are in no way a replacement for the energy and complex nutrient combinations found in whole foods.

Bottom Line: Stop Guessing.

Start Measuring and Managing...

Know the Calories You Burn

RMR: As you can see from the energy balance equation, your RMR number makes up the biggest part of the "Calories Out" side of the energy balance equation. If you are relying on a formula or estimate to give you this number, you might not be too far off from simply guessing. Knowing your real burn rate allows you to establish a calorie budget that works for you. It is also important to know your metabolism can change, sometimes significantly, as you lose weight. Having your metabolism measured throughout your weight management program will help you reach your goals without hitting frustrating plateaus or sacrificing valuable lean muscle.

Exercise: If you are currently active, add the formal exercise you do to this side of the equation. For the example provided in the exercise goals section at the end of Chapter 1: 5,000 steps per day or 2.5 miles would add about 325 calories to the burn side of your equation.

Lifestyle: We most always over estimate how many calories we burn during the day. Unless we are in jobs that require manual labor, most individuals only expend 150-300 calories daily due to their sedentary occupations. Use one of the many free diet and nutrition free apps to calculate these daily activity calories for you using the activity level that best describes you.

Use of Activity Trackers and Motion Sensors

There are many great new wearable technologies like the Fitbit, Fuelband and others that can help you. Also, apps that now sync with the motion sensors on smart phones to do the same to help keep you on track. Health monitoring with mobile technologies is becoming increasingly popular and there are many great new innovations in the pipeline to keep you motivated to move. One of the biggest areas of interest is how to use "gamification" to get you to move with rewards. Either way, you still have to make it happen and swallow that E-pill! I've included a list in my references section to help you choose which apps might help inspire you to make you accountable to take your fitness medicine!

Did you know? Just +/-100 calories every day over the course of a year equals approximately 10 pounds. Imagine shaving off just 100 extra calories a day through sensible diet changes and moving to expend just 100 calories more and you would be down 20 pounds of unwanted body fat by the end of one year. Getting a body in balance can be easy if you just start with simple consistent changes.

Smart Move:
Think you are already nutrition savvy?
Put your knowledge to the test with my online Nutrition IQ Test on the free Brainscape App (search "Weight Management") or look up:
Nutrition IQ Quiz

This link will also be provided in the Body in Balance resources section online.

Metabolic Syndrome
A Body Out of Balance

Is your Body Out of Balance?

The term metabolic syndrome is heard a lot these days in the popular media. Today we know more including the specifics of the syndrome, along with the link to obesity and poor health. I've defined it as a syndrome that relates to a body out of balance. Read on and I'll explain my balance position. First consider what may be happening to your own body using the "what" symptom checker on the left side with the "how" and "why" these symptoms may be revealing your own body may be out of balance.

The "What"	The "How and Why"
Fatigue	How has it become a disease?
Poor Libido	Why did it happen?
Pain	Why was it not prevented?
Trouble Sleeping	How do we reverse it?
Elevated Blood Pressure	How are my medications helping or hurting?
Elevated Blood Sugar	How can therapeutic exercise play a role?
Elevated Lipid Levels	Why hasn't my physician discussed diet alternatives?

What Is Metabolic Syndrome?

Metabolic syndrome is characterized by a cluster of symptoms: insulin resistance, hypertension, dyslipidemia, and obesity, all of which are well-known problems all with individual treatments. The problem in metabolic syndrome is the unique clustering of symptoms and it is a clear warning sign that the body is out of balance. It is now known that metabolic syndrome carries a high risk of heart disease, a fact nearly unknown to the general population. Type 2 diabetes is also frequently seen as a consequence. Prospective population studies suggest that metabolic syndrome is associated with approximately a twofold increase in the relative risk of cardiovascular disease and a fivefold increase in risk for developing diabetes.

Did you know? Currently it is estimated that approximately 25% of the U.S. population has metabolic syndrome!

What are the Signs Your Body is Out of Balance?

The most important risk factors of metabolic syndrome are abdominal obesity and insulin resistance, although you'll also see many of the symptoms under the "why" in the table as well as the other risk factors listed below.

Other risk factors are:

- Dyslipidemia (elevated triglycerides, small low-density lipoprotein [LDL] cholesterol particles and decreased high-density lipoprotein [HDL] cholesterol levels)
- Elevated blood pressure
- Elevated plasma glucose
- Atherogenic diet (ie, a diet rich in animal / saturated fat and cholesterol)
- Other conditions that may promote metabolic syndrome include aging, hormonal imbalance, and genetic or ethnic predisposition.

Our country's changing demographics, especially increasing age, are reflected in the increases of diabetes and metabolic syndrome but the toxic foods we choose to eat along with the sedentary lifestyles we lead are the largest contributors to obesity and this new "syndrome" created to classify it by the medical community. I have my own term for metabolic syndrome, I often get in trouble when I express it so simply but I am speaking the naked truth in this book so I will share it with you here as well. I believe the better term to describe metabolic syndrome would be to call it GOYA syndrome. You probably never heard of the term in medical circles but it stands for "**G**et" "**O**ff" "**Y**our" "**A**cetabulum"! You may have to look up acetabulum to get my physical therapy perspective, but when you do you'll find another three letter word "A_ _ "! actually fits in there better for GOYA emphasis and it so happens it is closely connected with the acetabulum too. Joking aside, if just get moving, learn responsible health strategies to help our Nation GOYA there will be no more epidemic of metabolic syndrome. In the meantime, the medical community needs to do a much better job at prescribing the magic E-pill for this syndrome, instead of multiple meds for high blood pressure, high blood glucose, elevated lipids and unbalanced hormones.

The Role of Obesity

Although there is no agreement on a single underlying cause, the driving forces behind metabolic syndrome are obesity and a sedentary lifestyle. These intricately linked conditions are responsible for an enormous burden of chronic disease and impaired physical function and quality of life.

Bottom Line

Sadly, metabolic syndrome (or GOYA) is a disease of modernity of urbanization, changes in food manufacturing including contaminating food sources with antibiotics, pesticides and untested genetic engineering, along with increased environmental exposure to plastics and hormone disrupting chemicals all in an effort to "help" increase societies convenience and mobility, and physical ease. It is sad that with all these "improvements" to help with convenience, they have come together to put a body further out of balance. As a result, our Nation is now fatter and sicker than ever before in history!

More on "GOYA" Syndrome and Prolonged Sitting

Here's the latest research on what happens with prolonged sitting:

Did you know? The body's metabolism drops 90% after just 30 minutes of sitting. The enzymes that transport bad fat from arteries to muscles slow down, and good cholesterol begins to drop.

Today, the average office worker sits for about 10 hours, first all those hours in front of the computer, sorting through e-mails, making calls or writing proposals — and sitting to eat lunch. And then all those hours back in the car to get home to sit again in front of the TV or surfing the Web.

According to the expert statement released in the British Journal of Sports Medicine, here's what you should be doing. Get up and stand! You should start standing up at work for at least two hours a day - and work your way toward four.

And more recent observational studies comparing workers who sit for long periods against those who sit for fewer hours have found that sedentary workers have more than twice the risk of developing type 2 diabetes and cardiovascular disease, a 13 percent increased risk of cancer and 17 percent increased risk of dying.

The World Health Organization estimates that 95 percent of the world's adult population is inactive, failing to meet minimum recommendations for health of 30 minutes of moderate to intense physical activity five times a week.

Experts acknowledge that evolving to routines with less chair time won't happen overnight, but the increased awareness about the need to move indicates that a longstanding health hazard can be combated with a simple commitment to moving.

That's a long answer for a growing number of workers who may have heard of the terrible health risks of prolonged sitting and been wondering whether they should buy standing desks or treadmill desks. While this may not be realistic in some settings, taking small breaks every 15 minutes or so to stand for a few minutes, (or GOYA!) will do wonders for keeping your body in balance.

As you move into the next chapter of Smart Moves Fitness, I'll be providing a measurement tool and simple exercise routine to correct your posture if prolonged sitting has already got you out of balance!

Smart Moves Fitness

Smart Moves Therapeutic Exercise Plan

This is my proven Smart Moves Quick Start Program I've been using successfully with clients for the past 25 years. Think of this as your Exercise Prescription, or "E" pill that I introduced you to earlier. These modules are the most effective way to combine cardiovascular conditioning with functional strength and core balance training. I am describing the background to the program here and I will provide links to videos and webinars for you to access once you complete and score your movement screen.

Background

My Smart Moves Quick Start program is a physical therapist designed therapeutic exercise program intended to take you successfully through the process of change to make you move better and restore muscle balance. The emphasis of this educational journey is to provide safe functional exercise strategies that will stay with you for the rest of your life. My goal in designing the guidebook is to provide the reader with the most effective therapeutic exercise combinations for change.

Within my comprehensive exercise program there are actually three versions:

Version 1: Provides a Home Fitness and/or travel training workout routine. This "no iron training" version can be done at home with minimal exercise equipment. This version begins with your own body weight then advances and uses a medicine ball or dumbbell, a stability ball, an exercise band, and an optional toning bar and step and builds on cardiovascular fitness using my walk/run progressions on in-between days.

Version 2: Provides "Smart Moves Circuits" to correct many of the movement screen imbalances found during the assessment. They can be performed at home and mostly use bodyweight but can be enhanced with dumbbells, bars and tubing.

Version 3: Is aimed at the advanced exerciser or athlete wishing to enhance their performance through a comprehensive series of multiplane sport specific exercises and stretches. This version provides a great introduction to some advanced training principles such as plyometrics, 10/20 (or Smart Moves Double Up) training along with the introduction to therapeutic PNF stretching protocols, and a few metabolism revving "HIIT" (High Intensity Interval Training) routine suggestions. This version is also ideal for people who have been following conventional exercise protocols and have found they've run smack into the dreaded plateau, the place where ongoing improvement becomes a challenge. The body has adapted to the workload it's being faced with and the necessity of adaptation ceases.

This program is not intended to be everything to everyone.

If you're erratic in your exercise habits, this is not for you. If you are about to begin Smart Moves, then you're someone who is serious and wants to made the exercise commitment.

This program is not intended to share every ounce of information the general public needs in order to improve the health of our nation. I continue to deliver that information in various formats, including our free monthly newsletter, but Smart Moves is built around several unique resistance training modules and progressions as well as smart nutrition principles that I have used in my private practice for over 25 years.

In order for anyone to succeed with lasting physical change, there is the primary foundational concept of Smart Moves Conditioning. I am referring to the all-important synergy of three elements:

- Smart Nutrition
- Moderate Aerobic Exercise and daily intentional movement
- A Concern for correcting muscle imbalances and revving up your resting metabolic rate

The primary discussion on aerobic exercise in this program will center around fitness walking and is described later in this chapter. Aerobic intensity can be judged by determining Target Heart Zone using the standard age related formula (220 - age x 70% - 85%), it can be judged by applying formulas that also incorporate your resting heart rate, or it can be judged by "perceived exertion." Very simply put, on the scale of 1 – 10, you should feel as if you're exercising at a 7 or 8. If you're too out of breath to carry on a conversation, you're working too hard.

WHY IS THE AEROBIC DISCUSSION SO BRIEF?

There are two reasons for brevity in addressing this topic:

1. There is a massive body of work in any library, on the web, and in the research labs related to aerobic exercise. I've also provided you with a chapter on aerobic exercise fundamentals as well as some Smart Walk/Run progressions in this section. We'll assume those who are ready to begin Smart Moves are already aware of the specifics of the aerobic element (referred to in the program as "Cardio").
2. The aerobic exercise is integrated into an overall program of strength, conditioning, and metabolic improvement and when it's applied as a part of the synergy, it is as simple as moving rhythmically for an extended period of time (although remember the word "moderate"). Your heart doesn't really know or care if you're running on a treadmill or doing laps around your neighborhood or in your backyard.

Many people mistakenly believe Aerobic Exercise is Fat Burning exercise. More accurately, aerobic exercise is movement that stimulates the cardiorespiratory system, and that's certainly a vital ingredient in striving for excellence. The reality is, making Smart Moves is the key, and with aerobic exercise alone there aren't any guarantees. You are capable of burning fat any time you're in an aerobic state. Aerobic means, "meeting the demand for oxygen." You're meeting the demand for oxygen when you drive, when you walk, when you watch TV, even when you sleep. Eat clean, follow the resistance training program Smart Moves is built around, and commit to the cardio time periods suggested and you can't help but succeed!

WHY IS THERE A NEED FOR SMART MOVES?

I developed this concept out of necessity and to have a reliable resource for my clients to follow upon discharge from physical therapy. I had worked with dozens of patients that left my clinic only to have to return after they became re-injured from falling off their program or worse going to a gym and trying "monkey-see monkey-do" exercises or classes that were not appropriate for them or advised by a questionable "trainer" with a weekend certification in "sports therapy". Yikes!!

Get Started!

Exercise is a must if any human being is going to facilitate a positive physical change. That's common knowledge, and some exercise is better than "no exercise." This program will also help you if you need an introduction to exercise. I've included background reading on aerobic and strength exercise in the chapters that follow so you have a good understanding of the importance of each component of fitness. I hope you'll take the time to learn more in this section and then take the tests included to begin to measure your progress. I've included the exercises for this section through links in the resources area so you can measure your current balance and then best learn and apply the corrective therapeutic movements.

David Dansereau

Aerobic and Strength Exercise

The Truth About Aerobic Exercise and Fat-Burning

By far the most popular questions I receive when I first start working with a new client that has come to see me for weight loss and toning is "How do I get rid of this belly fat?" or "What is the best exercise to target these love handles?"

The answer to this question is simple, there is no one exercise that will accomplish this goal. The fact is, stomach and thigh exercises (and their related machines) are not aerobic or fat-burning exercises. That's because they fail to meet one essential requirement. The activities don't last more than three minutes in continuous duration. Therefore, the exercise remains anaerobic. Why then do I "feel the burn" when I am using this equipment? The burning sensation is not fat being burned or "melted away." Instead, it's the muscles storage of lactic acid as glycogen (not fat) that has been used for energy during anaerobic metabolism.

Fat Burns in a Carbohydrate Flame

For activities more than three minutes, continuously, the body will continue to burn sugar (carbohydrate). However, it will begin to burn and breakdown the sugar in the presence of oxygen. This is known as aerobic glycolysis.

There is only one difference between the anaerobic glycolysis and aerobic glycolysis. Lactic acid does not accumulate in the presence of oxygen. In other words, the presence of oxygen inhibits the accumulation of lactic acid.

How Long?

The relationship between the "duration of exercise" and the "amount of glucose" used as a fuel depends upon the availability of oxygen. Oxygen plays a key role in the workings of the muscles' metabolic engines. With ample oxygen, muscles can extract all available energy from glucose in three to 20 minutes of moderate exercise. During this period of aerobic glycolysis the muscles and liver pour out their stored carbohydrate for use by the muscles.

However, the muscles and liver can only store and use a specific amount of glycogen before it will run out. Therefore, a person who continues to exercise moderately for longer than 20 minutes will need to find another source of fuel. At this point (after roughly 20 minutes) the body will begin to use less glycogen and more and more fat for fuel.

Think of the example of starting a fire. The kindling wood is the carbohydrate needed to ignite the fire and the larger and more plentiful logs are the fat and the main fuel to maintain the fire for an extended length of time.

Fat Supplies (almost) Unlimited Energy

Unlike the glycogen stores, which are limited, fat stores can fuel hours of exercise without running out. Body-fat is (theoretically) an unlimited source of energy.

Free Fatty Acids

Just as carbohydrate provides a basic usable form of energy in the body (glucose), so does fat. This usable form of energy in the body is called Free Fatty Acids (FFA). Fats taken in through the diet are first digested to produce fatty acids. After the fatty acids are absorbed they are converted to triglycerides. Triglycerides are the stored form of FFA. Stores of triglycerides are found in the adipose (fat) tissue and in the skeletal muscles.

Early in exercise the blood fatty acid concentration falls as the muscle begins to draw on the available fatty acids. But, if the exercise continues for more than a few minutes the hormone epinephrine is called into play. Epinephrine signals the fat cells to break apart their stored triglycerides and to liberate more fatty acids into the blood. After about 20 minutes of exercise the blood fatty acid concentration rises and surpasses the normal resting concentration and this is where fat cells begin to be mobilized for fuel.

Did you know? If you "front load" your strength training before you do your cardio, you tap your fat stores earlier where needed with your endurance training and give your muscles the preferred fuel the want (glucose/glycogen) for muscle building at the beginning of your workout too!

"How Long Do I Exercise?"

In general, the longer the duration of exercise, the greater the percentage of energy produced by fat. Keep in mind, however, that during the first 20 minutes the body is merely preparing to burn fat at a more efficient rate. After the 20 minutes the body will start to metabolize stored fat. Therefore, if you wish to burn fat by exercising, you should know that patient, persistent, consistent, moderate intensity training is the road to maximum use of fat and conservation of glycogen. A balanced consistent exercise plan is the preferred methodology to optimize a fat-burning metabolism. In other words, your personalized program should include building in exercise as much and as often as possible.

Muscles Are Trained Fat-Burners

The more time spent during aerobic activity, the more trained the muscles will become in fat metabolism. Trained muscles can burn fat more efficiently and require less glucose, even during strenuous exercise.

After physical activity has ceased, "fat-burning" may continue at an accelerated rate for some time. Some reports suggests that fat metabolism remains elevated for at least six hours after completion.

Another report suggests there is increased fat use 24 hours after an hour-long aerobic session. The body's adaptation to strenuous and prolonged aerobic exercise burns more fat all day, not just during the exercise. In other words, consistent exercise for more than one hour will most likely raise an individual's resting metabolic rate, which means you consistently burn more fat even while not exercising. This phenomenon is called **EPOC** (excess post-exercise oxygen consumption) and it is a process of recovery of oxygen after the body has completed intense bouts of work that raises your metabolism. Here's my "real life" example below:

```
My Metabolic Monitor Test
Rhode Island Hospital Lab

Date of test 17-Apr-1991

Height   5'11"
weight   170
Age      23
Predicted Basal Metabolic Rate:  1870 kcal/24hr

Measured Result:                 3050 kcal/24hr

Difference from predicted:       + 63%
```

The results above were from a metabolic test I did at RI Hospital while I was still a (young!) dietetic intern. I had an opportunity to get under a metabolic hood while a technician monitored my results. What is significant about the date of this test is that it was less than 48 hours after I had run the Boston Marathon. My running weight then was lean for my frame at just 170 pounds, but the power of EPOC had me still burning over 3,000 kcal at rest which you can see was over 63% higher than my predicted rate based upon age, height and weight alone. I still remember trying my best to walk around the floors and stairs of the hospital that day. Boy, was I sore!!

"How Intense is Intense?"

As well as duration, intensity plays an important role in the efficiency of fat-metabolism during exercise. In general, the percentage of energy contributed by fat diminishes as the intensity of exercise increases.

Fat can only be broken down in the presence of oxygen. Oxygen serves as the catalyst that enables proteins and enzymes of the body to burn fat during an exercise metabolism.

The heart and lungs can provide only so much oxygen — so fast. When muscle exertion is so great that the demand for energy outstrips the oxygen supply, the body cannot process oxygen fast enough. Therefore the body cannot burn fat. Instead, it reverts back to anaerobic metabolism and burns more glucose.

Oxygen Debt

When your body reverts back to this anaerobic metabolism, it has incurred an oxygen debt. Oxygen debt occurs when you become out of breath. When intensity of exercise is so great as to incur oxygen debt, aerobic metabolism cannot sufficiently meet energy needs.

Slow Down

Muscles must instead draw more heavily upon their limited supply of glucose. When this happens, glucose is spent rapidly. As a result, fragments of glucose molecules accumulate in the muscle tissue and cause fatigue. This is why, if you exercise intensely, you may have to stop or slow down to "catch your breath" (replenish your oxygen supply). By slowing back down your body will once again rely upon aerobic metabolism.

Therefore, exercising with too much intensity will inhibit the body's ability to burn fat. Keep intensity in check by engaging in moderate, low-intensity aerobic activity. This includes activities where energy demands do not exceed the available oxygen, and fat can supply much of the energy, permitting glycogen to be conserved.

Target Heart Rates

The most effective method of monitoring exercise intensity is to check your target heart rate (THR). The target heart rate gives an <u>approximation</u> of where your heart rate should be at a certain percentage of its maximum capacity in order to burn fat.

An individual exercising at 75% of his/her maximum heart rate will be exercising in an aerobic fashion. It's also helpful to establish a THR Zone. This is done by taking the maximum heart rate (220 – Age) and multiplying that number by both 65% and 85%. These numbers will establish the upper and lower limits of your zone. By keeping your heart rate between these two numbers during exercise your body will burn fat.

Dividing the Target Heart Rate and Target Heart Rate Zone numbers by 6 will determine 10 second guidelines for easier heart rate checks during exercise. This can be accomplished by counting your pulse either on your neck or wrist with your first two fingers for 10 seconds.

Remember, exercising at an intensity greater than the upper target heart rate zone limit (220 – Age x 85) requires more energy consumption than the body can handle (working too hard). It will start to break down glycogen to keep up. Exercising below the lower limit (220 – Age x 65) is not working hard enough. The body will not need to engage its aerobic pathways. In both cases, the body's ability to burn fat becomes <u>less efficient</u>.

There is a basic "rule of thumb" concerning aerobic exercise. You should exercise at an intensity that allows you to carry a normal conversation. If you are out of breath, you are in oxygen-debt and not burning fat.

"How Often Should I Be In My Target Heart Rate Zone?"

For the person interested in maintenance or moderate reduction of body fat, 3 to 4 days a week may be all the body requires to achieve these goals. However, for the individual interested in making a noticeable reduction in body-fat, then, 5 to 6 days per week of 45-60 minute aerobic conditioning may be necessary. The final determinant of how much cardiovascular activity is required to reach your goal, however, cannot be answered in these pages. The final decision comes from how your body reacts to the <u>amount</u> and <u>frequency</u> of aerobic exercise you perform during your program. Some individuals may lose their body-fat with 4 days at 45 to 60 minutes while others may require 6 days a week or even twice a day to reach their goal.

Get All Your Muscles Involved...

To maximize efficient fat-burning metabolism, your activities should involve as many muscle groups as possible. The more muscle mass required to perform, the more energy required to feed that exercise.

Activities such as walking/jogging/running outdoors or on a treadmill, are effective fat-burners as long as you're in your target heart rate. These are efficient activities because you are supporting your own body-weight in an upright position and your upper body is free to move.

The same holds true for aerobic type classes. However, be sure to stay within your THR during these classes. Even though you may participate in an hour-long class, actual cardiovascular activity may last only 35 to 40 minutes.

Equipment such as the stair climber will be a little less efficient if you hold on to the rail. This is because the upper body is not moving freely to burn as much energy. The stationary bicycles will even be less efficient because the seated positions do not burn the same amount of energy as the person supporting their own weight, unless of course you opt for an all-out high energy spin class where you are constantly being cued to come up out of your seat and stand to pedal.

Efficient Fat-Burning

We can summarize that the human body uses available fuel sources in a very efficient way. Utilization and efficiency is dependent upon timing. Knowing this, it's obvious we should use efficiency to our advantage. Individuals interested in performing both anaerobic activities (to improve and/or increase their lean muscle mass) and aerobic activity (to burn body-fat) should perform these activities in the proper sequence to obtain maximum results.
Performing anaerobic activities before aerobic activities will enable the exerciser to utilize their fresh stores of available ATP and glucose for their anaerobic activities when needed. Also by using a portion of the stored ATP and glycogen prior to aerobic exercise the body may start to burn fat sooner than the standard 20 minute guideline, thus increasing exercise efficiency.

Fat-Burning Summary

For efficient metabolism of fat during exercise:

- Exercise at least 30 minutes and up to 45-60 minutes
- Exercise as often as possible (5-6 days per week, even twice a day)
- Exercise in your target heart rate zone (65 to 85%) of your maximum).
- Perform anaerobic activities prior to aerobic activities to optimize your workout performances.
- Exercise consistently and in moderate intensity

Building A Balanced Body through Strength Training

There are countless books on weight-training, body-building and general fitness conditioning. To cover all aspects would be an impossible task. Instead, the focus of this chapter is on the important basics of weight-training.

It also will outline the principles behind resistance training for improved overall health and fitness.

"Muscular fitness" is paramount to achieving your particular weight-management goal. That's because long-term, credible weight-management can only be achieved through a systematic weight-resistance training program – of almost any kind.

These programs can be designed for a variety of purposes such as power lifting, body building, rehabilitation or just simple muscular conditioning and toning like rowing a boat, paddle boarding, yoga, Pilates, etc.

You may already be engaged in a weight-training program. On the other hand, you may not feel a need for weight-training. Many people have preconceived notions and stereotypes about weight-training. As a result, they have no interest in this type of exercise program at all. It is a HUGE mistake! Remember the example I gave you earlier on the research with sarcopenia (muscle loss) with aging? It is never too late to start strength training!

Training for All Reasons

Strength and weight-training is important for fat-burning. The most apparent effects of weight-training (resistance) are increased strength and muscular endurance. These gains often are accompanied by an increase in the size of muscle fibers. This is known as muscular hypertrophy.

Sometimes an increase in muscular size is due to an increased number of muscular fibers. The increased number of fibers results from what is referred to as longitudinal fiber splitting. It's generally accepted, however, that increases in muscular size is a result of an increase in the size of existing muscle fibers.

Weight Training and Fat-Loss

A structured weight-training program is the most effective way to increase and improve the quality of muscle. This should be of particular importance to anyone interested in achieving optimal fitness and health. And, of even more important to anyone interested in losing body-fat.

Why is weight-training so important to the reduction of body-fat? To answer that question, refer back to metabolism.

Muscle requires energy to function. Fat can only be burned in the muscle. Therefore, the more muscle mass you have, the more fat you can burn. Improving your muscular condition will improve your basal metabolic rate

(BMR), thus, increasing the body's ability to burn calories.

Anaerobic or Aerobic?

Since most weight-training activities last less than 3 minutes in duration, (regardless of actual workout time), weight-training is an anaerobic activity. This means that the primary fuel sources will be either ATP or glucose. The aerobic (oxygen/fat) fuel system does NOT come into play. Therefore, fat is NOT burned as a fuel source during weight-lifting activities. However... even though weight-training does not burn fat, it does increase the body's fat-burning potential.

Women Should Lift Hard Too

The thought of increased muscular size may not appeal to some. In the past, women were reluctant to weight-train for fear of becoming too muscular or bulky. For most women, however, muscular gain is not as great as in men, even when they make the same relative gains in strength.

A study that compared muscular size between men and women, demonstrated that "muscular hypertrophy in women as a result of weight-training programs will certainly not lead to excessive muscular bulk or produce an undesirable effect" when done with a balanced approach in mind.

Methods of Weight Training

Various methods of muscular contractions have been used to improve muscular strength and endurance. Here are a few methods with explanations and benefits.

Static (Isometric) Training – Isometrics involve muscular contractions performed against fixed, immovable resistance. The muscle develops tension, but does not change length. Static exercises are widely used in rehabilitation programs. Isometric training can be used effectively to counteract strength loss and muscle atrophy, especially in cases in which the limb is temporarily immobilized. This method of training would be compared to flexing one's bicep or pushing against a wall and holding the contraction for 6-10 seconds. A major disadvantage of static training is that the strength gains are specific to the angle of the joint used during the training or contraction. Therefore, to increase strength throughout the range of motion, the exercise needs to be performed at a number of different joint angles.

Isokinetic Training – An isokinetic contraction is one in which maximal tension is developed throughout the full range of joint motion. Increases in strength, power and muscular endurance are acquired by mechanically controlling the speed of the movement with special isokinetic equipment. The availability of this type of equipment is either limited and/or not available to many and is often only found in sports or rehabilitation therapy settings.

Dynamic (Isotonic) Training – Dynamic (isotonic) weight-training involves both eccentric and concentric contractions of a muscle group performed against a constant or variable of resistance. During a concentric contraction the muscle will shorten as tension is developed (e.g. curling a weight with the biceps). Just the opposite occurs with an eccentric contraction. The muscle lengthens as it develops tension (e.g. setting the weight back down with the biceps). Dynamic training is the most familiar kind of contraction since it is the kind used in all lifting activities. There are three important concepts used to describe and classify dynamic weight-training programs — repetition, set and repetition maximum.

Learning the Lingo

Reps & Sets

A repetition is one actual movement of an exercise through the full range of motion (i.e. one push up, one pull-up, one squat, etc.) A set is a done consecutively without rest.

One of the most common ways to calculate and measure an individual's progress and strength is to perform repetition maximums for a given exercise. And then, record the progress over time in a written journal or workout log.

A repetition maximum is the maximum amount of weight an individual can lift a given number of times before fatiguing. For example, if an individual could do a bicep curl with 50 pounds for 8 repetitions and no more before fatiguing, that weight (50 pounds) is an eight-repetition maximum load.

Principles of Weight Training

There are four principles that should form the basis of most weight resistance programs. For best results training should involve overload and progressive resistance with careful attention going to arrangement of the program and the specificity of its effects.

Overload Principle

Muscular strength is most effectively developed when the muscle or muscle group is overloaded – that is, the muscle is exercised against resistance exceeding those normally encountered. If an individual is accustomed to bench pressing 150 pounds on a regular basis then, a resistance of 155 pounds or more, is required for muscular strength and growth to occur. The use of resistance that overloads the muscle stimulates the physiological adaptations that lead to increased muscular strength and development.

Overloading a muscle during exercise is your way of telling the body that the current muscular strength and development is not enough. Therefore, it needs more.

An overload can be applied to the muscles two ways:

- Application of a resistance or weight greater than can be lifted for one repetition (strength).
- Forcing a muscle group to repeatedly lift a load or weight over an extended period of time (endurance).

For example, if an individual can only curl 55 pounds 2 times, then they have two options to improve strength and development.

- The individual can force their bicep muscles to lift 60 pounds one to two times (strength) or,
- The individual can train to lift 55 pounds 4 times (endurance). Either way the muscle is forced to overcome a resistance to which it is not accustomed.

Progressive Resistance Principle

Throughout a weight-training program, the work load (overload) must be increased periodically to continue muscle overload. A gradual increase in resistance or maximal repetitions will ensure further improvement in strength or endurance. It is important this increase be gradual. Too much too soon may injure the musculoskeletal system.

Nonetheless, it's important to understand that a muscle must encounter progressively increasing overloads. Many individuals will continue to exercise with the same resistance (weight) at the same number of repetitions for weeks... even months. By exercising against a resistance that is encountered time after time with no overload, the muscle will adapt and no gains will occur.

The Principle of Arrangement of Exercise

A weight-training program should include exercises for all major muscle groups. For optimal efficiency during weight-training, the exercises in a weight resistance program should be arranged so that the larger muscle groups are exercised before the smaller muscles. Smaller muscles tend to fatigue sooner and more easily. Therefore, in order to ensure proper overload of larger muscle groups, they should be exercised first. The larger leg muscles should, for instance, be exercised before the smaller arm muscles.

Specificity Principle

The development of muscular fitness is specific to the muscle group that is exercised, the type of contraction and training intensity. This simply means, that to increase the strength of the elbow flexors (biceps), exercises must be selected that involve the concentric and eccentric contraction of that muscle group. This also applies to increasing strength for improving a specific sports skill (i.e. soccer kick baseball throw, football technique, gymnastics, etc.).

This means that not only must the specific muscle be exercised for improvements, but the exercises will be most effective if the pattern of the movements is simulated. This "motor-skill" specificity not only applies to specific skills or movements, but also to overall conditioning of muscles. For example, the professional skier who is in excellent condition to ski, may not have the strength or endurance to run a marathon (and vice-versa). Although in both activities the same muscle groups are used, the movement patterns they produce are quite different.

Applications

Now that we have identified the types of weight resistance exercises and the appropriate principles that accompany them, we may continue on with some guidelines and direction as to setting a specific program to meet your needs.

Remember that all individuals are different and may respond accordingly to different types of weight training programs. Every individual must assess their own goals and fitness levels to determine what type and intensity of a program may be right for them. Those individuals with chronic heart conditions or other musculoskeletal conditions may want to consult their physician before starting a weight training program.

Success and results will ultimately come down to consistent trial and error of the appropriate principles and techniques of weight training to determine what works for you.

I've provided Smart Moves Walking and Running Progressions in in this book along with a Smart Movement Screen you can try at home before you get started to identify general muscle imbalances before you begin. I strongly suggest you score well on the movement screen before you advance to any higher level (running) progressions. You can't build fitness on dysfunction so you'll need to identify muscles needing attention first and then restore balance with some simple corrective exercises!

David Dansereau

Smart Movement Screen

How to Measure if Your Muscles are in Balance

My Smart Movement Screen is a quick system for a simple and quantifiable measure of evaluating your current movement abilities. This is not a comprehensive assessment but rather a quick way to "flag" which muscles need immediate attention. I've used this on professional athletes, models, actors as well as kids and seniors as a starting point in their rehabilitation. Can you guess who does the best on this test of all the groups I mentioned? You would think it would be athletes, right? That would be the incorrect answer. Kids generally have the best scores when I measure them against adults. This is because they have not generally had the time to develop muscle imbalances from compensating for old injuries or prolonged occupational postures like adults expose themselves to daily.

Every day, out-of-shape people attempt to regain fitness, lose weight, and become more active and they often jump in "cold turkey" into a bootcamp style workout routine like Crossfit or oftentimes a P90x type similar DVD series. They assume if they just move more, they will start to move well. Unfortunately, without proper screening and corrections they will just get better at moving poorly for longer periods of time or with larger amounts of weight or at greater speeds. As problems arise like aches, pains and injuries, some will change equipment or listen to a friend and try a new class, some pop a pain pill or two and try to press on, others simply quit only to try over again the next year. I often see this group of individuals in my office only after they have become injured. They'll report to me they felt something "pull" in their back when they were flipping a tire, or something "tighten up" in their shoulder when they were swinging ropes, or heard a "pop" in their hip when they were doing side-kicks. In each case, they didn't even have the range of available motion in those joints to complete that movement pattern even one time, never mind doing it repeatedly under a load with added weights and high velocity.

You can't build fitness on dysfunction so this self-assessment will help identify areas of your body's musculoskeletal balance that may need attention before you take on your exercise plan. Think of this screen as a muscle system test, much like blood pressure measurement is a way of screening at the surface for the health of your cardiovascular system.

<u>Goal of this Module:</u> To identify physical imbalances and weaknesses through a series of Functional Movement patterns.

<u>Outcome:</u> Exercises are prescribed based on test results to correct weakness or imbalance.

What is Your Smart Movement Score?

Find out with this quick and easy at-home test based on the more comprehensive 7 item PTC Smart Movement Screen assessment which we adapted from Gray Cook, co-creator of the Functional Movement Screen.

<u>Our word of warning: Prepare to be humbled.</u>

What you'll need: Masking tape, a 4-foot dowel (a broomstick works), and a doorway (32" to 36" wide)

How to do it: Follow the directions for each fitness screening. If you can do the move correctly, and without any pain, you pass that test and get a "3" score. For each screen that you flunk, add 5 years to your current age to get your "movement age."

Score Sheet (lowest score 1 / highest score 3)

MOVE	Test 1 (day 1)	Test 2 (day 15)	Test 3 (day 30)
Deep Squat			
Hurdle Step			
Inline Lunge			

Notes:

The Tests

DEEP SQUAT

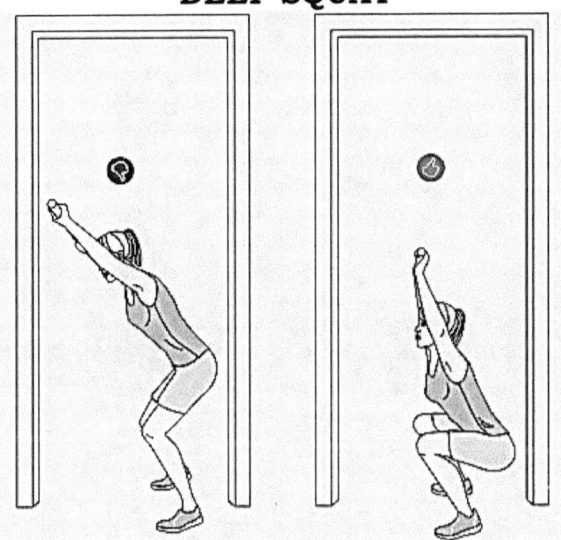

Place strip of tape on floor in middle of door frame. Stand with feet shoulder-width apart, toes pointing straight ahead and in line with tape. Hold dowel overhead. Descend into full squat. Return to starting position.

How to Score:

You pass if... You can lower into a deep squat (thighs parallel to floor) while keeping dowel overhead, toes forward, and heels on floor. Give yourself a "3" on the score sheet.

You fail if... You feel pain, your heels lift, the dowel tips forward, or you can't lower into the full squat (signs that you're lacking hip and ankle mobility). Give yourself a "2" if you could do the move almost to full range with small compensations mentioned here. Score "1" if pain stopped you from trying or you were fearful of the movement and wouldn't try to complete.

HURDLE STEP

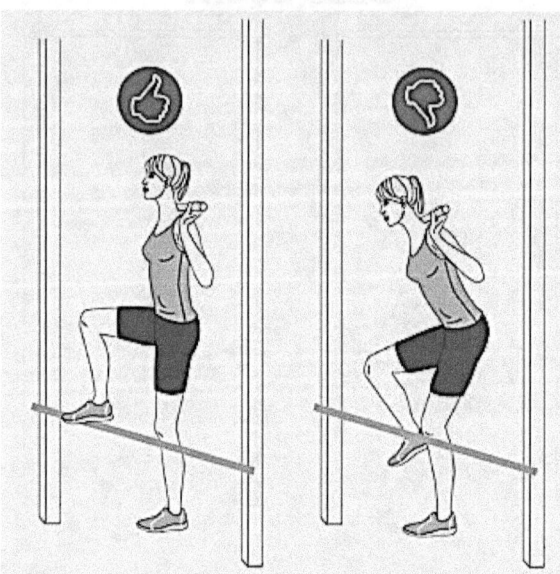

Stretch strip of tape across doorway so it's in line with bump just below kneecap. Stand with feet hip-width apart, toes beneath tape, and dowel behind neck and across shoulders. Balancing on left foot, bend right knee and lift sole of right foot over tape. Hold 5 seconds. Lower foot back to start. Repeat on opposite side.

How to Score:
You pass if... Your lifted foot doesn't touch tape and chest remains lifted. Give yourself a "3" on the score sheet.
You fail if... You feel pain, your shoulders tip forward, your foot touches tape, or you sway side-to-side (signs that your hips are tight). Give yourself a "2" if you could do the move almost to full range with small compensations mentioned here. Score "1" if pain stopped you from trying or you were fearful of the movement and wouldn't try to complete.

INLINE LUNGE

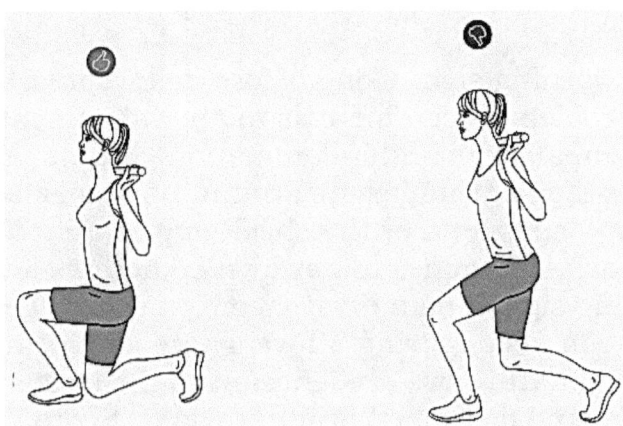

Place strip of tape on floor. Stand on tape in split stance, one leg a few feet in front of other leg; hold dowel across shoulders. Slowly lower back knee to touch tape behind front foot. Pause, then return to start. Repeat on opposite side.

How to Score:
You pass if... Your feet remain on tape and point straight ahead throughout movement. Upper body remains straight and still. Give yourself a "3" on the score sheet.

You fail if... You feel any pain, your torso tips forward, you lose your balance, or you cannot easily bring your back knee to the floor (signs that your ankle and hips joints are lacking mobility and that your core is weak). Give yourself a "2" if you could do the move almost to full range with small compensations mentioned here. Score "1" if pain stopped you from trying or you were fearful of the movement and wouldn't try to complete.

David Dansereau

Why do I get a "1" if I can still do the test but with pain?

Pain is a warning sign. Long before pain represents a chronic problem, it can alert us to poor alignment, overuse, imbalances and inflammation. We usually listen to all the other warning signs around us-smoke alarms, computer virus alerts or the check-engine light in our cars- but when it comes to our own bodies, we act as if the warning sign of pain is an inconvenience. We cover it up so we can keep moving. If we ignore pain's natural self-limiting nature, we are ignorant to the lessons our own smart well developed brain provides. Score the test appropriately so you can listen to your body and accurately measure your progress over the next 30 days. I've provided you links to some corrective movement exercises in the resources section.

Modern technology and marketing pain management is in on the cover up

Technologies offer ways for us to compete and get through life with pain. Temporary solutions have become standard practices especially in sports. Wraps, braces, drugs and new high tech tapes were originally developed in the athletic arena to allow athletes to get through just one game or event. Now these high tech band aids are accepted as normal playing gear and using braces and tapes over topical creams and numbing gels are part of the athletes game. The terrible part is parents are buying into these solutions for their injured and overused kids joints with no concern for the long term effects on their bodies. "*I just need to get* him/her *back on the field so they don't miss the tournament*" is the most common excuse I hear when a parent would come to visit me with a child in pain and distress.

This same mentality is playing out in our older sedentary society as well. Recently, I watched a commercial you may have seen that was selling "medicaid/medicare paid for braces" for just about every joint in your body direct on TV. "Just have your doctor fill out this form and we'll bill it to your insurance and even cover the shipping all free-simply give us a call!" No wonder no one is swallowing the "E" pill when they can get high tech band aids delivered to their door without so much as getting off the couch. In reality it is a sad reflection on how marketing pain management has gone way too far.

Smart Walk-Run Progressions

The Importance of Warm-up and Stretching

- Proper warm-up and stretching helps reduce injury and improves performance.
- The first 5-7 minutes of a run/walk should be easy in order to gradually warm-up muscles.
- Stretching is more effective after the run.
- Key areas: hamstrings, calves, lower back, hip region, quads.
- Do not bounce!
- Do not stretch beyond the point of tension, but not in pain.
- Hold each stretch for 30 seconds – do two sets of stretches minimum
- Stretching can be done every day.
- The cool down should consist of 3-4 minutes of easy walking after the run or walk, and should be done every time.

<u>Getting Started Checklist</u>

- Get a good pair of running shoes from a running specialty store.

- See a sports physical therapist if there are any previous or current injuries that may impact your performance.

- Review the five training profiles and pick one that fits your goals, current training status, and find availability to train.

Body in Balance

Here's the Progressions

Training Profile # 1- Walker

Training Profile # 2- Transitional Walker/Runner* (Pole Training)

Training Profile # 3- Beginner Runner

Training Profile # 4- Intermediate Runner

Training Profile # 5- Advanced Runner

*Run? YES! I know what you may be thinking. "I have not run in years!" "I'll get hurt!" I will perhaps put your fears at ease with a question. When did you lose the ability to run? Think about it, you never lost it you just became conditioned to the fact that you became deconditioned! You probably ran often as a child, and with great confidence too! Think about this, if you only make your pace a bit faster than you are going today, that is running to you. Faster than you walk to get the mail is a good place to start.

Did you know? One of the best predictors of risk of falling as we age is average walking speed. Several studies have been replicated which show that when maximum walking gait speed drops below 1.6 miles per hour the incidence of falls increases dramatically. My theory is stay fast and strong for long!

This program can be done at your own pace from a "no fitness" baseline (Profile #1) up through using the advanced progression (Profile #5) that could take you right up to competing in your own ½ marathon. Imagine that! This is the same routine I designed for myself and used to restore fitness to run the Boston Marathon safely after my stroke.

Training Profile # 1: Walker
Current Status: No structured exercise at all
Goal: To walk race
Walking days per week: 3-4

	Monday	Tuesday	Wednesday	Thursday	Friday	Saturday	Sunday
Week1	Walk 15 min at BP	Off	Walk 15 min at BP	Off	Walk 15 min at BP	Walk 2 miles	Rest
Week2	Walk 20 min at BP	Off	Walk 20 min at BP	Off	Walk 20 min at BP	Walk 2.5 miles	Rest
Week3	Walk 25 min at BP	Off	Walk 25 min at BP	Off	Walk 25 min at BP	Walk 3 miles	Rest
Week4	Walk 30 min at BP	Off	Walk 30 min at BP	Off	Walk 30 min at BP	Walk 4 miles	Rest
Week5	Walk 35 min at BP	Off	Walk 35 min at BP	Off	Walk 35 min at BP	Walk 4.5 miles	Rest
Week6	Walk 40 min at BP	Off	Walk 40 min at BP	Off	Walk 40 min at BP	Walk 5 miles	Rest
Week7	Walk 45 min at BP	Off	Walk 45 min at BP	Off	Walk 45 min at BP	Walk 6 miles	Rest
Week8	Walk 50 min at BP	Off	Walk 30 min at BP	Off	Easy 1 mile	RACE DAY	Rest

*BP- Brisk Pace
*min- Minutes
See following pages for introduction of walking into running program

How to begin a Smart Running Program
(If you have not been running at all)

Start with 10 total minutes of jogging (use Training profile #2 to help you build up to 10 minutes of jogging). It takes the joints much longer to adopt to running than the heart, lungs, and muscles so don't go crazy with too much enthusiasm at the start. Injury prevention is the most important component to a running program.

HERE IS A SUGGESTION OF HOW TO BEGIN:

					total jog time:
Week1	walk or cross-train 15 min.	jog 5 min.	walk 5 min.	jog 5 min.	10 min.
Week2	walk or cross-train 15 min.	jog 7 min.	walk 5 min.	jog 7 min.	14 min.
Week3	walk or cross-train 15 min.	jog 9 min.	walk 5 min.	jog 9 min.	18 min.
Week4	walk or cross-train 15 min.	jog 11 min.	walk 5 min.	jog 11 min.	22 min.
Week5	walk or cross-train 15 min.	jog 12 min.	walk 5 min.	jog 12 min.	24 min.
Week6	walk or cross-train 15 min.	jog 14 min.	walk 5 min.	jog 14 min.	28 min.
Week7	walk or cross-train 15 min.	jog 16 min.	walk 5 min.	jog 16 min.	32 min.
Week8	walk or cross-train 15 min.	jog 17 min.	walk 5 min.	jog 17 min.	34 min.

The walking portion could be replaced with cardio, cross-training on a bike, elliptical, stair master, cross-country, etc.

- Third week could just walk or cross-train on other days
- Once you build up to 40-60 min per day, three days a week; stay at this point and check in with your physical therapist (that's me) to discuss advancing to the next program level.

David Dansereau

Training Profile # 2
Transitional Walker/Runner with Pole Training

Telephone pole training is an interval training technique which can be used by advanced runners but it also quite effective for new runners who are transitioning from a walking to running program. Either way, the concept behind pole training is the same, it utilizes a sequence of intervals to improve performance. Interval training is alternating intensity of activity during a workout to increase aerobic capacity and help burn more calories. While classic interval training is done on a track, telephone pole training is a good alternative for runners on the road. Telephone poles, or utility poles, are used as landmarks along the running route. With the goal of building both speed and endurance, runners purposefully vary their speed and recovery intervals from pole to pole.

Here's How:
The Basics
- Runners who can't make it to the track for interval training or speed work can get the same results on the road. Rather than using laps on a track to define intervals, runners use the distance between telephone or utility poles. After warming up and stretching, find the nearest telephone pole. Start at a comfortable pace and maintain your speed until you reach the next telephone pole. Then reduce your speed (from jog to fast walk) until you reach the next pole. Speed up again and jog to third pole. Now return to a brisk walk to the next pole and repeat the cycle. Follow these repetitions with a brief cool-down period, and you'll have completed an interval training session.

- If you check your heart rate after following a 1:1 (jog:walk) ratio and it is above a safe range for your fitness level, allow more recovery time between intervals by changing to a reduced intensity such as 1:2 ratio with two telephone poles recovery time between jog intervals.

Interval Training
- Interval workouts can significantly improve performance. In fact, interval training is standard in many runners' training programs for everything from slashing 5-kilometer times to improving marathon results. At the same time, interval training can work for every fitness level from beginner to elite athletes. According to the Mayo Clinic, workouts that include regular bursts of intensity build endurance and burn more calories than lighter workouts. Interval training is also easier on muscles than workouts with sustained higher intensity.

Benefits

Telephone pole training can be done along any route with utility poles alongside it, making an interval workout possible just about anywhere. This technique can also provide lower impact on your joints while you improve your weight/bodyfat ratio and develop better running form. At the same time, adding a telephone pole training component to your regular walking/running route can help combat boredom, forcing you to stay alert and on task from pole to pole. Focus on getting to the next pole, rather than completing an overall distance, to make a workout less routine.

Variations

There are countless, customizable variations to the basic interval outlined above. For example, you can switch to a more intense jog-run-sprint-walk routine (1:1:1:1) to improve running time. One popular version uses the poles to create a stair-step routine where you speed up from one pole to the next, then slow down between the next two poles, and then accelerate for a longer distance at the next pole--passing a pole in between without changing speeds. Another version includes slowing down between poles and then repeating the cycle but adding a pole to each acceleration period. If you find the distance between two poles is too short you may choose to vary speeds by every other or every third pole.

Training Profile # 3: Beginner Runner

Current Level: Runs less than 8 miles a week or no running.
Goal: To run the entire race without walking.
Run days per week: 3
Cross-Training days per week: 2

	Monday	Tuesday	Wednesday	Thursday	Friday	Saturday	Sunday
Week1	Walk/XT 25 min/Off	Run 15 min	Walk/XT 25 min/Off	Run 15 min or Off	Run 15 min or Off	Rest	Run 3 miles
Week2	Walk/XT 25 min/Off	Run 18 min	Walk/XT 25 min/Off	Run 18 min or Off	Run 18 min or Off	Rest	Run 3.5 miles
Week3	Walk/XT 30 min/Off	Run 21 min	Walk/XT 30 min/Off	Run 21 min or Off	Run 21 min or Off	Rest	Run 4 miles
Week4	Walk/XT 35 min/Off	Run 25 min	Walk/XT 35 min/off	Run 25 min or Off	Run 25 min or Off	Rest	Run 4.5 miles
Week5	Walk/XT 35 min/Off	Run 30 min	Walk/XT 40 min/Off	Run 30 min or Off	Run 30 min or Off	Rest	Run 5 miles
Week6	Walk/XT 40 min/Off	Run 33 min	Walk/XT 40 min/Off	Run 33 min or Off	Run 33 min or Off	Rest	Run 5.5 miles
Week7	Walk/XT 45 min/Off	Run 35 min	Walk/XT 40 min/Off	Run 35 min or Off	Run 35 min or Off	Rest	Run 6 miles
Week8	Walk/XT 40 min/Off	Run 25 min	Off	Run 15 min or Off	Off	RACE	

*XT- Cross- Train (Elliptical, Bike, Swim, Smart Moves Circuit, etc.)
*min- minutes

David Dansereau

Training Profile # 4- Intermediate Runner

Current Training Status: 15-20 miles per week
Goal: To run for "x" desired time.
Run days per week: 4
Cross-Train days per week: 1-2

	Monday	Tuesday	Wednesday	Thursday	Friday	Saturday	Sunday	Total Mileage
Week1	3mi MP 5xS	30-40 min XT 10min hard @ end	4-5 mi MP	IT (see guide) 4 x 400	30-40 min XT or Off	6 mi	Off	16mi
Week2	3.5mi MP 6xS	5-40 min XT 12min hard in middle	4.5-5 mi MP	5 x 400	30-40 min XT or Off	6.5 mi	Off	18
Week3	3.5mi MP 6xS	35-40XT 15/mid	5mi MP	6 x 400	30-40 XT or Off	7 mi	Off	21
Week4	4mi MP 7xS	40-45 XT 15/mid	5 mi MP	3 x 800	30-40 XT or Off	7 mi	Off	22
Week5	4mi MP 7xS	40-45XT 15/mid	5.5 mi MP	4 x 800	30-40 XT or Off	7.5 mi	Off	23
Week6	4.5mi MP 8xS	45-50XT 15/mid	5.5 mi MP	5 x 800	30-40 XT or Off	8 mi	Off	24.5
Week7	4.5mi MP 8xS	45-50XT 20/mid	6 mi MP	5 x 800	30-40 XT or Off	6 mi	Off	26
Week8	5mi MP 8xS	40-45 XT	5 mi MP	3 mi easy 4xS	2 mi easy 2xS	RACE		15

*mi- Miles *MP- Moderate paced run (You can carry on a conversation, but are slightly winded) *S- Strides 10-12 second accelerations focusing on form *IT- Interval Training (Read How To Design an Interval/Pole Training Plan) *XT- Cross training (elliptical, Bike, Swim, Smart Moves Circuit, etc.)

Training Profile #5- Advanced Runner

Current Mileage- 30 + per week
Run days per week- 4-5
Cross-Train days per week- 1-2

	Monday	Tuesday	Wednesday	Thursday	Friday	Saturday	Sunday	Total Mileage
Week1	5mi MP 8xS	60min XT 20min hard in middle	6mi MP	ITraining (See Guide) 6 x 400	30-40min XT or Off	8-10 mi	Off	30
Week2	5.5 MP 9xS	60min XT 20/mid	6.5 MP	8 x 400	30-40 XT or Off	10 mi	Off	33
Week3	6 MP 9xS	60min XT 20/mid	6.5 MP	4 x 800	30-40 XT or Off	10 mi	Off	36
Week4	6 MP 10xS	60min XT 20/mid	7 MP	4 x 800	30-40 XT or Off	11 mi	Off	40
Week5	6.5 MP 12xS	60min XT 20/mid	7 MP	5 x 800	30-40 XT or Off	12 mi	Off	30
Week6	6.5 MP 12xS	60min XT	7.5 MP	6 x 800	30-40 XT or Off	12 mi	Off	42
Week7	7 MP 14xS	60min XT	7.5 MP	7 x 800	30-40 XT or Off	10 mi	Off	44
Week8	6 MP 10xS	4mi MP	Off	3 mi easy	2mi easy 2xS	RACE		

*min- minutes
*mi- miles
*MP- Moderate pace
*S- Strides 10-12 second accelerations focusing on form
*ITraining- Interval Training (see tipsheet)
*XT- Cross training (elliptical, bike, swim, etc)

Note: PDF versions of all these profiles are available for download in the online resources area. Many of the tables had to be reduced in size to fit in this book format therefore the image quality may not be the best.

The Importance of the Long Run/Walk
(if you eventually want to train for an endurance event)

- The single most important component of the training program is the Long Run/Walk.

- The Long Run/Walk prepares the muscles, ligaments and joints for the long-duration exercise.

- The long run trains the muscles to efficiently use energy.

- The long run builds self-confidence and mental toughness.

- The long run burns a tremendous amount of calories.

- This schedule may be adjusted to meet the individual needs.

- Some long runs may feel easier than others, based on the given day.

- The day before the long run should be a day off, or an easy workout.

- The long runs become the dress rehearsal for the actual race.

- Pace of the long runs should be slightly slower (30-60 sec/mile) than the typical weekly run.

- Get a good night sleep the night before a long run.

- The meal the night before the long run, as well as the breakfast the morning of the long run, are very important to a successful long run.

Injury Prevention is the Key:

- 80% of running injuries are caused by too much of an increase in mileage.
- The cardiovascular system adjusts to the stress quicker than the joints.
- Joggers/runners should increase their total weekly running/walking amount by no more than 10%.

Tips

- Get a good pair of running shoes and change them every 400-500 miles.
- Run or walk on soft, flat surfaces whenever possible. Treadmills are fine.
- If you cannot take more than a couple of days per week of impact, cross-train on bike or elliptical trainer to increase fitness level.
- Maintain or achieve ideal bodyweight to minimize joint stress.
- Stretch regularly, and add strength training to your program.

What do I do if I become injured?

- Ice area: 15-20 minutes several times per day (frozen peas work well).
- Elevate injured part while icing.
- Rest (at least at first)
- Contact your coach to develop a game plan to continue the program.
- Analyze problem for probable cause:
- What did I do differently in training?
- Was there a big mileage jump?

- Was there a significant increase in pace?
- Were my shoes inappropriate? Wrong model?
- Was there a change from treadmill to road work?
- Cross-train on non-impact cardio.
- Determine plane to return to full program, return to run/walking very slowly.
- Possible physical therapy/orthopedic consult may be needed.

What pain is OK?

- General muscle soreness.
- Slight joint discomfort after workout or next day, that is gone in 24 hours.
- Slight stiffness at beginning of run/walk that dissipates after first 10 minutes.

What pain is not ok? (You should not train!)

- Pain that keeps you awake at night.
- Pain that is evident at the beginning of the run/walk then worsens as you continue.
- Pain that changes your stride.

Smart Brain Fitness

If you can take IQ tests over and over again, study them, get help figuring them out, and learn how to do them quickly and well, your score will improve. Does this mean your brain is now more fit? Some would argue that this is not really increasing intelligence, but indeed it is. Experiences that challenge the brain's cognitive abilities raise intelligence–real intelligence. IQ tests, while certainly not a great indicator of how well someone will do in life, are a pretty decent indicator of memory, problem solving skills, and other cognitive functions. Obviously, an abundance of these skills is helpful.

A better idea than taking IQ tests over and over again is to do some other brain teasers, learn a language, and learn to constantly exercise your brain. Constantly strive to keep learning!

Combine these mental push-ups with the right diet, a fitness program that pumps oxygen to your brain cells, and a few brain supplements, and your focus will be sharp while your cognitive ability will improve significantly

The more you practice using your brain in various, challenging ways, the better you will get at using it. The better you take care of your brain's health, the more efficiently and easily it will work, and the longer it will work as well.

David Dansereau

How your Brain is Connected to Your Gut

Your brain is very connected to your gut. We have a symbiotic relationship with every microbe living inside us, and the highest concentration of microbes is in our gut. In addition, parasitical influences, like candida running rampant throughout our bodies (that consume a sugary standard American diet) keep our gut out of balance and cause us to crave more junk food, and stress our intestinal health. Typical foods that feed candida include concentrated sugars (corn syrup, sugar, agave, fruit juices, etc.) as well as flours, white breads, rice and pastas. The candida fungus has been identified as a possible cause and a definite contributor to depression as well. Getting your intestinal health up to par is the most important first step in increasing your intelligence. Healthy gut = healthy body = healthy brain. Refer to the chapter on greens of you need an attack plan here for candida.

Restoring your gut flora or good bacterial health is necessary for balanced hormones. Gut bacteria produce 90% to 95% of our serotonin, the key neurotransmitter responsible for regulating mood. We need bacteria to assimilate B vitamins, which are essential to the function of the nervous system and the brain. Without enough B vitamins, we can't concentrate well.

Gluten in those with sensitivity is also believed to lead to an overabundance of candida and a host of other problems in the gut and the whole body which directly affect the brain's ability to function. GMOs are very suspicious and foreign to our guts too, so clear them off your plate to protect your brain cells!

Brain Boosting Herbs

If you're looking for a quick boost to help you, there are lots of herbs and other things you can do right away. If you're looking to increase your cognitive abilities over a period of time, and enjoy life with a clear head and all the focus you need, then the first step for most people is to kill the candida and balance the gut, so don't skip that section above!

Ginseng

Ginseng is a well-known stimulant that can reduce stress, increase focus and memory, and raise metabolism and energy levels.

Sage

Sage has been shown to improve memory. Sage is being investigated as a potential treatment for Alzheimer's disease.

Rosemary

Rosemary stimulates the pituitary gland, which produces the HGH (human growth hormone) needed to regulate weight and look younger. It also improves memory, along with a host of other benefits.

Ashwagandha

This herb is to Ayurvedic medicine as ginseng is to Chinese medicine. People use ashwagandha for improving cognitive ability and it treats many other health problems from infertility to inflammation.

Vitamins, Minerals and Fats Our Brains Need

A deficiency in any one of the following nutrients can lead to brain health issues. Even less than optimal levels can impair cognitive function.

B Vitamins

B vitamins are the vitamins of the nervous system and they are needed for the numerous functions critical to every cell in the body. B vitamins are essential for hormone production, stress management, and the metabolism of carbohydrates, proteins and fats. B vitamin deficiencies are not uncommon, and lead to many physical and mental illnesses. Anyone suffering from an inability to concentrate, PMS or other hormonal issues, insomnia, depression, or virtually any other mental health issues should reach first for B complex.

Vitamin C

Vitamin C is more than an anti-oxidant and necessary vitamin for fighting infections and viruses, it is necessary to synthesize the neurotransmitter norepinephrine. It also helps the body flush heavy metals such as iron and copper from the brain.

Vitamin D

Normal brain development and function is dependent on vitamin D. Deficiencies have been proven to impair cognitive abilities.

Vitamin E

Vitamin E is essential to maintain the integrity of cell membranes. Among other symptoms, a deficiency in this vitamin manifests in neurological symptoms including injury to sensory nerves and impaired coordination and balance.

Calcium

The brain requires calcium for secretion of neurotransmitters. The body maintains a specific level of calcium in the blood at all times, pulling calcium from the bones, if the level in the blood drops too low. So deficiencies generally affect bone health, not the brain.

Iodine

The thyroid requires iodine to produce its hormones, which are used in the myelination of the central nervous system. It is also critical in the development of the brain, therefore deficiencies during pregnancy can result in various neurodevelopmental deficits from mild cognitive deficits to mental retardation.

Iron

Iron is essential for proper development of the brain cells that produce myelin and for the synthesis of neurotransmitters. An iron deficiency during fetal development can cause permanent learning and memory deficits; childhood deficiency also causes cognitive impairment.

Magnesium

Magnesium is essential for metabolic reactions required for brain function. Deficiency results in neurological and muscular symptoms.

Selenium

Selenium is required for antioxidant enzymes in the brain and other tissues.

Zinc

Zinc plays a role in neurotransmission as well as catalytic, structural, and regulatory roles. Deficiencies can cause congenital malformations, deficits in learning, and other deficits including attention and learning.

Choline

Choline is another essential nutrient needed for myelination of nerves, neurotransmitter synthesis, and cell membranes and other structures of the brain and nervous system. Deficiency is related to cognitive defects.

Antioxidants

Your brain uses a lot of oxygen, and therefore, it is highly susceptible to free radical damage. This is why antioxidants are critical brain boosters. They protect brain cells by neutralizing free radical damage and preventing premature brain cell aging. Anthocyanins, the antioxidants that are found in berries, have been found to be particularly beneficial to the brain. See the color coding your kitchen section for more help on choosing high antioxidant foods.

The Right Fats are Good For Our Brains

Numerous studies have proven that eating a balanced diet with healthy fats, and/or a fatty acid supplement with omega 3s, are imperative for all brain functions. It's no wonder, since the brain is about 60% fat (if you exclude water, which makes up about 70%). DHA is a fatty acid chain that is one of the major building blocks of the brain, critical for optimal brain health and function. Of the many fatty acids that benefit the brain and offer noticeable cognitive improvement, DHA is the most significant. Balanced healthy fats are also needed to properly assimilate B vitamins. When you talk about food for the brain, cold-water fish top the list due to the fat content. Fish like salmon, sardines, trout, mackerel, and cod contain significant amounts of omega-3 fatty acids and essential amino acids in proteins that build healthy brain cell membranes and improve cognitive function.

Other great foods for the brain (especially if you're vegetarian or vegan) include:

- Avocados, pumpkin seeds, various nuts, and other oils containing healthy fats along with vitamin E
- Leafy greens and cruciferous vegetables provide antioxidants and brain defending carotenoids
- Berries give the brain vitamin C, create healthy connections between brain cells, and protect brain cells against free radicals with antioxidants.
- Turmeric's active ingredient, curcumin, detoxifies the brain.

- Cayenne can wake you up like nothing else, rushing blood to the brain. Cayenne is a great supplement to take with other remedies.
- Ginger protects the brain and has some of the same effects as cayenne, as far as waking up the senses and increasing blood flow.
- Pretty much all produce nourishes the body and therefore the mind.

Use It or Lose it

Our brain works much like the rest of the body in that it is a "use it or lose it" organ. If you don't use your brain enough, your cognitive abilities suffer. People who really think more than the average person, like scientists and professors, are less likely to suffer from Alzheimer's and other degenerative diseases of the brain.

Studies show that learning a new language increases intelligence measurably. It's not just languages though. Learning anything complicated that takes lots of time and practice, that uses the brain in many different ways, will have a noticeable effect on intelligence. If speaking another language isn't in the cards, learning to play a musical instrument, mathematics, or learning computer languages can offer the same benefits.

Learning how to develop websites, for instance, is an excellent way to exercise the brain. One way I helped my brain heal after my stroke for example was by learning HTML and CSS (a new language to me) to build websites.

Body in Balance

There are also countless apps and websites with daily brain-teasers and exercises. Most of us know that reading increases our intelligence, but processing a variety of information has a greater affect than just reading fiction or a single other genre. All reading, whether it be fiction, magazine articles, blog posts, or historical, has benefit and can work our brains in different ways. Just like "cross training" improves overall body fitness, try reading different topics to "cross train" for your brain fitness!

Exercise itself is huge for brain health! Being physically fit has been show to help with concentration. Exercise regulates proper hormone production, and exercise is the best way to take a break from an arduous brain task.

Be sure to keep taking those free IQ assessment tests when you can, too. What better way to raise your IQ than to practice taking various different IQ tests? There are also lots of toys and games like the classic Rubik Cube. If you really want to turn your boost your brain, playing with brain teasers, puzzle toys, crossword puzzles and the like should be a hobby. Collect them and use them on a regular basis.

Breathe Right

Take deep, slow breaths. Breathe so that your abdomen expands with each breath and your ribcage compresses with each exhale to get more oxygen to your brain. See my unique meditation technique I used to help heal my brain in the chapter on breathing.

Drink Plenty of Water

Most people are chronically dehydrated. Coffee and sodas are only making it worse. Our brain is made up of 75% water. Sometimes when concentration seems impossible and the day feels like it's spiraling out of control, chugging a few cups of water with a bit of lemon can change perception and get things back on track.

Maximum Brain Function Regimen

Obviously, I eat well, typically consuming lots of produce with beneficial fats, enzymes, antioxidants, and all the other nutrients my body needs. But sometimes I need a boost. If I am tired, having trouble focusing, can't figure something out, or am in need of some brain help for any reason, I tend to go for a huge salad with plenty of greens, nuts and seeds and healthy brain fats like from avocados. I spritz it up with a mix of apple cider vinegar, tumeric, lemon, ginger and olive oil (and sometimes some cayenne) and this brain boost of greens and healthy fats get my brain back in order fast!

Conclusion

The most important and significant thing you can do to increase your concentration and other cognitive abilities right away without making any lifestyle changes is to breathe right, eat clean, drink plenty of plain filtered water, and do regular bursts of oxygen driving exercise, like a few sets of overhead reach squats that I show you in the Smart Movement chapter.

Resource

If you need help with finding great salads and other plant based recipes I suggest you grab a copy of the *New American Plate* cookbook by the American Institute for Cancer Research. I've included a link in the resources section to this guide. This book has by far the best soups and salads recipes compiled with powerful brain boosting and cancer fighting ingredients.

David Dansereau

Improve Posture Flexibility and Breathing

Try Yoga and Meditation

Setting aside 10-15 minutes to practice mindfulness or meditation will fortify a sense of calm throughout your nervous system, mind, and brain. There are many different types of yoga and meditation. "Meditating" doesn't have to be a sacred or new-crazy "religious" experience. I suggest that you do more research, visit a meditation center if you can, and fine-tune a daily meditation practice that fits your schedule and personality. Below are some basic principles to get you interested.

Background Why it Works

There are many ways to improve the quality of your life, but one that you may not have thought of is that of meditation. Some don't believe it can offer benefits but there is one thing that meditation and yoga can definitely provide for you: the ability to relax and get in touch with your breathing. Simply put, here how meditation works on the body. Any type of meditation will reduce anxiety and lower cortisol levels. Simply taking a few deep breaths engages the vagus nerve which triggers a signal within your nervous system to slow heart rate, lower blood pressure and decreases cortisol. The next time you feel yourself in a stressful situation that activates your 'Fight-or-Flight' response take 10 deep breaths and feel your entire body relax and decompress.

Here's How it Works:

Yoga is a great tool for both exercise and relaxation. Both meditation and yoga have been shown to provide improvements for those that are in need of stress relief. And, when you learn how to do them effectively, it takes minutes a day to wash away your stresses. I have personally benefited from increasing my body awareness through these strategies but also have educated clients on how to do the same by incorporating some poses in with their more traditional therapeutic exercise plans.

So, how could this fit into your own lifestyle fitness plan? It's simple. You need to spend ten minutes each day, usually before breakfast, quietly meditating or doing yoga. Ten minutes per day is all that it takes to see significant improvement in your overall well being, including your posture and flexibility, while at the same time "calming" your mind.

When you take into account all the things that you are doing in the morning you may not think you have time. But, again, invest the time for a couple of weeks and you are sure to see the improvements quickly and they will not be such a demanding time taker.

You can learn how to do either meditation or yoga (or both if you like) easily. Some people are familiar with it enough that they can learn how to do is through at home study. It's often a better solution, though to learn with others through a professional.

Get together with a friend and take a class at your local recreation center or your community college. You'll find that once you learn the technique you can do the process on your own, easily. If you say you have no time to go to a class, try picking up a few DVD's at your local library. In a big rush? Then you really need to make the time to try this. Go on YouTube and search meditation and you'll find plenty of good resource videos at your fingertips.

It's funny to look at it this way, but one of the things that has promoted the spread of yoga in the west, is the same thing that can sometimes prevent someone from truly exploring it and therefore experiencing its health benefits. This thing is variety.

Sometimes when there is only one of something – such as one idea, or one language, or one anything – it's hard for that thing to spread outside of those who abide by it, agree with it, or simply want it to continue existing.

Yet when there are multiple ideas and concepts, the chances of it spreading increase; there are just more people out there who will be able to access it, talk about it, and indeed, make it a part of their lives.

What does this have to do with yoga? Well, there are many different types of yoga; and the reason for this, as we initially discussed, is that yoga isn't a religion; it's an approach to being alive. As such, it's very agile and flexible (no pun intended!) and carries well across cultural, country, and religious boundaries.

Thanks to its diversity and different facets and types, yoga has spread very swiftly through the western world over last 110 years or so; and is spreading faster now than ever before (many western companies will now pay for yoga classes as part of an enhanced health benefits program).

Yet this very diversity has led to some confusion; and people who have been exposed to one kind of yoga might accidentally think that they've seen it all. This is more worrisome, of course, when one has been exposed to a kind of yoga that – for whatever reason – they did not like, or perhaps, weren't quite ready for (just as how some people might turn away from a fitness program if they aren't in the right frame of mind to see it through).

So if you've experienced yoga, or seen it on television, read about it in a newspaper, or overheard a friend or colleague talk about it, then please be aware that there's a very good chance that you haven't been exposed to all that is out there. I've included a link in the resources section on how you can access a kickstarter yoga workout to try.

David Dansereau

Smart Moves Nutrition is about Eating Clean

How to Eat Clean

Eating clean is a process of eliminating poor quality foods from your diet and replacing those items with the clean burning fuels the cells in your body need every day to repair and perform at their best. In the chapters that follow you'll find tips to help you eliminate the junk and processed foods as well as ideas to help you stock up on the top foods to fuel your activity. I've included background chapters on carbohydrates, fats and proteins so you have a better understanding of these macronutrients and the important role each play in delivering complete balance nutrition. So let's get started.

Commit to Breakfast

Eat breakfast to benefit your waistline, your metabolic rate, and your heart

One of the first things that people do when they want to lose extra weight is eliminate a meal or skimp on a meal and try to replace it with a mindless "weight loss" shake or commercial breakfast bar. The meal that most often gets short changed is breakfast.

Make no mistake- possibly the biggest fatal flaw most individuals make to interfere with their fat loss efforts is skipping breakfast.

I go over this topic in great detail in my Smart Moves Guidebook as well as how Americans are getting duped by commercial weight loss centers and marketers who pitch meal replacement drinks and bars, as well as "smart" waters and "energy" drinks.

Instead, start your day off right. It is true, breakfast is THE most important meal of the day. It is designed to get your metabolism up and running. It can actually help you in the long run with burning more calories effectively due to the thermic effect of food (TEF) as well as help you maintain blood sugar and "save calories" later in the day.

While many people use artificial stimulants like coffee or soda to get them going in the morning, you should consider complete whole food nutrition as your real energy source.

David Dansereau

Here's some recent evidence to support my position on the value of breakfast:

Skipping breakfast could increase your chances of gaining weight and developing heart disease, according to new research from the United Kingdom.

In summary: The researchers fed young healthy women breakfast for two weeks, then had them skip breakfast for two weeks, while monitoring their calorie intakes, blood cholesterol and insulin levels. They discovered that when the women skipped breakfast, not only did they eat more during the day (an average of 100 calories more each day), they also had 10% higher blood levels of insulin, 9% higher total cholesterol and 17% higher low-density lipoprotein (LDL) or "bad" cholesterol. The researchers conclude that skipping breakfast may increase a woman's risk of heart disease by raising LDL's, decreasing insulin sensitivity and triggering weight gain.

American Journal of Clinical Nutrition

Think that 100 extra calories a day is not that significant? Well, consider that those little 100 extra calories over the course of 1 year translate into adding approximately 10 pounds of extra fat on the scale.

Need more proof?
In a study of 2,831 people, researchers at Harvard University found that those who ate breakfast every day were 44 percent less likely to be over weight and 41 percent less likely to suffer from insulin resistance-a precursor to diabetes-than those who had no a.m. meal.

Why?

Skipping breakfast only trains your metabolism to slow down and you lose the energy revving benefit from the TEF. No food-no TEF. Also, nutrition is essential to metabolism and your nervous system has preferred sources of fuel. Your brain can only use glucose or blood sugar as fuel and it needs this glucose especially first thing in the morning upon waking from essentially a 7-12 hour overnight fast. In this case the body's first choice for fuel is stored glycogen (blood sugar) to help keep its nervous system operating. At this point, if food is not present, the body turns to protein, and breaks down lean muscle mass, to feed its basal metabolic rate.

Many dieters incorrectly skip breakfast because they believe the body will burn fat as its alternative source of energy. <u>This is wrong</u>. At this stage fat stores are of no use to the nervous system and the body does not have the enzymes to convert fat to glucose. Bottom line: If you want to keep burning your muscle as fuel, keep skipping breakfast and your metabolic rate will suffer making fat loss impossible.

"America runs on" poor breakfast choices

I added the "poor breakfast choices" to the beginning of a popular commercial jingle used by Dunkin Donuts which boasts the "America Runs on Dunkin" slogan they've crafted to advertise their products. I have to comment on this because I heard my son recently singing this catchy jingle as he ate breakfast one morning. I had to at least try to change the lyrics a bit for him because, well, his dad is a nutritionist after all. [Anyway, I digress from my personal sidebar and continue...]

By eating breakfast, I don't mean the drive through franchises or express coffee shops. In fact, anything from a foam cup or a paper bag should be off limits at least for the next 30 days while you are restoring your body to balance.

Consider this little "on the go" breakfast example at Starbucks:

A medium latte and blueberry scone will set you back 740 calories and a whopping 21 grams of artery clogging saturated fat !!

I added this fact just so you wouldn't think I was ranting exclusively on Dunkin'.

I don't assume you will give up all "on the go" eating, but I use the example above to show just how bad choices like this easily can set you way off target from your fat loss efforts. Remember, we are learning skillpower here to regain a balanced body!

If you need a quick online meal planning resource to see if your diet is making the grade, try my online meal planner PTCMAP. If you give my book a good review I'LL GIVE THIS TO YOU FOR YOUR VALUABLE FEEDBACK!. Learn more in the resources section.

Either way, I've given you several smart breakfast choices below to help you get started with better morning fuel selections. These are just a few morning meal suggestions you can quickly add to your breakfast skill power set and give your metabolism a boost.

Smart Breakfast Choices

Sustained Energy "Slow Burn" Carbohydrates

I know this is controversial, but yes, I am suggesting slow burning carbs are a wise choice for breakfast, especially for an active body that has been engaged in exercise and needs to refuel brain cells and muscle glycogen to support the next workout. Be sure to choose wisely and select products with whole grain as the first ingredient or better yet make your own morning breads and cereal options with recipes found in the *New American Plate Cookbook*. Look for whole wheat, whole rolled oats, brown rice, barley, or some of the more exotic grain mixtures such as spelt, triticale and amaranth. Also look for the whole grain label on these products as a quick indicator of the amount of whole grains used in the product and stay clear of any brands that are sneaking in extra sugar to add flavor, especially high fructose corn syrup!

Here's a few breakfast suggestions on ways to include ancient whole grains as a sustained-energy carbohydrate choices. These naturally nutrient-rich foods are easy to find on supermarket shelves but if you have concerns for gluten sensitivity or have been scared into believing all grains are "bad" then you have plenty of "gluten-free" options available today as well. I discuss this controversial topic later in the carbohydrate section as well as give my opinion on the currently popular *Grain Brain* and *Wheat Belly* diet books that have incited a grain hysteria (when the real issue just may be portion distortion). Stay tuned!

The following are a few simple ways to incorporate whole grains into your breakfast. Choose ancient grains, or non-hybridized varieties of:

1. Whole grain organic sprouted breads and rolls: Add nutrient rich goodness to toast or to build your favorite whole grain breakfast sandwich.

2. Organic whole grain hot cereals: Choose steel cut

oatmeal and other multigrain hot cereals to help kick your energy level into high gear and help stabilize blood sugar levels.

3. Organic whole grain cold cereals: Make a morning parfait with layers of crunchy cereal, fresh fruit, and berries.

4. Low-fat whole grain homemade muffins: Bran muffins are just the beginning. Try whole wheat with blueberries or oatmeal with bananas and nuts. Be careful here- the best choice is to make your own. Many commercial muffins are no more than a donut in disguise and can pack even more calories and saturated fat. Again, see the recipe book I mentioned for great options here.

5. Organic whole grain pancakes: Multigrain, spelt or buckwheat pancakes are a nutrient dense morning treat with fresh or frozen strawberries, local honey or greek yogurt.

6. Whole grain pasta: Check out what's new in the pasta aisle and find varieties made with ancient whole grain goodness. Small portions can be tossed in with scrambled eggs or egg whites to give more power to your breakfast.

POW!-My Favorite Breakfast Blast

One of my favorite breakfast meals is what I refer to as my "Power Breakfast". Here's how to make it:
1. Use 1 cup precooked quinoa (or use whole grain (leftover) pasta), warmed up in a skillet with ½ TBS olive oil
2. Scramble in 3 egg whites
3. Toss in 1TBS wheat germ,1TBS ground flax,1TBS fresh parmesan or feta cheese
4. For more flavor toss in a few raisins, dates or figs if you prefer
5. Add salsa on top upon serving

Heat till eggs are done and POW! - more energy than you'll know what to do with that will carry you through even the busiest of mornings!!

I performed an analysis below to demonstrate how "re-thinking" breakfast might give you a new way to target your fat loss efforts. Even by using regular pasta (because many of my clients tell me "they just can't use whole wheat") you still get 10 grams of fiber and a real energizing balanced meal with less than 2 grams of saturated fat and 415 calories. Now, compare that with the Starbucks example...

Our Most Vital Nutrient

Water-The most overlooked nutrient

<u>Bottom line:</u> If you are skipping this section because you *"just don't like plain old water"*, you should know this fact. Your hydration status can positively or negatively affect your fat loss efforts. Incredible as it may seem, water is quite possibly the single most important catalyst in losing weight and keeping it off.

Although most of us take it for granted, and probably only drink half of our daily requirement, water may be the only true "magic-potion" for permanent weight-loss.

Read on to understand this important fact and why most of us walk around dehydrated and sabotage our efforts at burning excess fat.

Here are some fluid facts to consider:

Water makes up about 60-70% of the body weight of adults. Your body can survive over a month without food, but within around a week without water it will die. The reason for this is water performs so many necessary functions in your body's metabolism which are essential for sustaining life. Let's look at some of these roles which rank <u>water as one of the 6 essential nutrients for life</u>.

- As the primary fluid in your body it serves as a solvent or catalyst for minerals, vitamins, amino acids, glucose and many other small molecules, including fat from your diet and helping burn the excess bodyfat stored on you! Without water, digestion, absorption and proper utilization of the fuel from food and stored energy (your fat cells) is impossible.

- Water aids your body to help keep your core temperature from rising to dangerous levels. Essentially, water is your body's natural cooling system.

- Water is part of the transport mechanism by which nutrients and waste products are carried throughout your body. Water is an active participant in the chemical reactions that keep you alive. Not only does it fill virtually every space in your body in and between cells, it also helps form the structures of molecules like proteins and glycogen.

- The big mistake many people make even when they are carefully regulating their diets, is lack of attention to their body's fluid needs. Granted, foods are the energy source by which the body produces fuel for exercise. But did you know that only around 25 percent of that energy is actually used for mechanical work? The other 75 percent or so is released as heat. This is the energy which causes your body to get warm or heat up during exercise. To get rid of this extra heat and protect your core temperature, your body starts sweating. As the sweat evaporates, your blood and your body are cooled. If you could not cool off with water from your body, you would quickly succumb to heat stress and illness. If your body does not have enough fluids to spare to sweat efficiently, evaporation won't occur and dangerous consequences can result. Studies show that thirst is not a good indicator of your actual fluid needs because fluid changes occur very quickly.

How water can influence Fat Loss

Water can suppress the appetite naturally and helps the body metabolize stored fat. Studies show that a decrease in water intake will cause fat deposits to increase, while an increase in water can actually reduce fat deposits.

Why? Your kidneys can't function properly without enough water. When kidney function is reduced, some of the work load is taken on by the liver. The liver's primary function is to metabolize stored fat into usable energy. If the liver has to do some of the kidneys work, it can't function at its optimal capacity. As a result, it metabolizes less fat. More fat remains stored and weight-loss/fat-loss stops.

The best way to overcome water retention is to give the body more water. The body will then release the stored water. Diuretic medications and weight loss schemes that intentionally dehydrate the body offer only temporary relief of water retention. Your body will perceive this as a threat to survival and will slow down metabolism, try its best to save fat stores and burn lean tissue, all while trying to hold on to every spare drop of fluid.

If you have a constant problem with water retention, excess salt or sodium in your diet may be the issue. Consider the physiology here: the more salt you consume the more water your body will hold. Your body holds water to dilute the salt because your body can only tolerate so much sodium. Drink more water to flush your system as sodium passes through the kidneys. In addition, try looking at how much salt is in the foods you are eating. There are now many free and paid apps that can show you instantly how your diet rates for sodium intake and can make suggestions on ways to reduce your intake.

Water helps to maintain muscle by giving it the natural ability to contract and by preventing dehydration. Remember, as I stated earlier, your muscles are primarily made up of water.

Consider the following example to illustrate the need for water in the body.

A 150- pound man carries approximately 45 quarts of fluid in his body. A 120-pound woman carries about 36 quarts of fluid. With these two people, if they are inactive and live in a cool to moderate climate, the man will lose about three quarts of fluid a day and the woman about two and a half quarts a day through perspiration and excretion. In a hot and humid climate, the same two people, Mr. and Mrs. Inactive, will lose even more water. Mr. Inactive can lose more than 10 quarts and Mrs. Inactive more than eight quarts in one day. If it's really hot and humid, they could lose more than two quarts of water in an hour!

What are some of the warning signs of dehydration?

Generally the average person is not 100 percent hydrated to begin with. Add a warm climate, as we demonstrated with Mr. Inactive, and it can spell dehydration, especially if Mr. Inactive were to begin an exercise program. Scientists define dehydration as fluid loss greater than just one percent of body weight. Here are some early warning signs to look for:
- Fatigue
- Flushed skin
- Light-headedness
- Loss of appetite
- Heat intolerance
- Dark urine with a strong odor

Monitor yourself for early signs of dehydration by taking these steps:

1. <u>Check the color of your urine.</u> It should be light in color to clear with little odor. If it is a golden or deep color with a strong odor, you are dehydrated.
2. <u>Weigh yourself without clothing before and after exercise.</u> Any weight lost during exercise is fluid loss and should be replaced by fluids as soon after exercise as possible. Use the general rule: *"A pint is a pound. For every pound lost during exercise, you lose a pint (2-cups) of fluid. Replace each pound lost with 2-cups of fluid.*
3. <u>Watch for muscle cramps</u>. Sweat loss and dehydration can disrupt the balance between the electrolytes potassium and sodium, leading to cramps. Adequate fluid replacement is necessary to restore electrolyte balance.

4. <u>Dehydration is cumulative</u>. Your body unfortunately cannot re-hydrate itself. If you fail to re-hydrate on numerous occasions, you will become increasingly dehydrated and begin to suffer from the early symptoms of dehydration mentioned.

Can water help improve performance?

Certainly. Even though water is calorie free, it is a wise investment to use it to enhance your fluid intake. Without it, performance would drop significantly. When water is drawn away from working muscles, blood volume is decreased so the heart must pump harder to supply the same amount of energy.

Consider what would happen with Mr. Inactive our 150-pound man if he lost 2 percent of his body water (six cups of water, or 3-pounds): His physical and mental performance would drop by 20 percent. If he lost 4 percent of his body water (twelve cups, or 6-pounds), his performance would drop by 30 percent, and he would be at risk for heat exhaustion. So you can see that fluids are important to sedentary individuals as well as active exercisers. But how much fluid should you drink?

Am I drinking enough?

All sedentary adults need a minimum of eight to ten cups (two quarts) of fluid every day. Exercisers need this minimum amount plus they need additional fluids to replace fluids lost through exercise. Again, do not rely on your sense of thirst to help signal you to drink. Your sense of thirst is diminished during exercise, so don't depend on it to prevent dehydration. Once you are thirsty, you are already dehydrated.

<u>Smart Moves Tip</u>: In addition, the overweight person needs one additional glass of water for every 25 pounds of excess weight.

Here are some hydration tips for active individuals:

Before exercise
Drink eight to sixteen ounces (one to two cups) of fluid two hours before exercise to make sure the body is well hydrated. This will also allow you time to eliminate any excess prior to exercise. About 15 to 30 minutes before exercise, drink an additional four to eight ounces of fluid (one half to one cup). This will give you fluid in your system available to replace sweat losses.

During exercise
Try to drink from four to eight ounces every 15 to 20 minutes during exercise. This might seem difficult at first, but with practice as part of your exercise routine, your body will adapt to taking fluids. In fact, the fuller your stomach with fluid, the faster it will empty and become available to your body. If you are an athlete, it is important not to wait until the day of a competition to try this. Instead, try immediately to make this a part of your routine.

After exercise
Try to drink at least eight to sixteen ounces of fluid (one to two cups) or more depending on how much weight you have lost. Replace any fluid you have lost using the *"pint equals a pound"* guideline mentioned.

30-60 Minutes before a Meal

Drink eight to sixteen ounces of fluid (water!) to help satisfy sense of fullness and be sure you aren't mixing signals of actually being thirsty with signs of hunger. This also helps you get in a scheduled routine to ensure proper hydration.

At Mealtime:

Sip water, don't drown your food!

Try adding a squeeze of lemon to your plain water or a small dash of apple cider vinegar to help you neutralize your stomach. Only sip during meals so that the needed acids are available to break down your food.

Put Smart Energy In

Start by knowing how many calories you consume

Most people I coach in nutrition simply have no idea how many calories they eat each day. This is the equivalent of writing checks without knowing how much money you have in your account. If your funds are not there to cover your checks, they bounce. If your calories aren't there to cover your nutrition needs, your body "bonks". I usually reserve the term "bonk" to describe what happens to athletes when they have not planned their pre-competition meals well enough and they "hit the wall" and can't continue to compete. In this example of basic every day meal planning however, most individuals who have not figured out their nutrition budgets end up "bonking" at the end of the day by making poor food choices.

Weight management success is a simple matter of balancing your calorie budget- or the calories you eat with the calories you burn. The calories you eat can be tracked easily so you know how much you are consuming. There are many free and paid online apps, but however you do it, you need to know what is in your current nutrition account first.

I still encourage keeping a physical journal when you are beginning to understand your nutrition and exercise habits. It is proven that the physical act of writing goals down (as well as your food and exercise habits) on paper makes a better imprint in your brain. For now, use some of the links in my resources page to get a clear picture of how many calories are in your energy balance checkbook.

Do I need to record my goals forever?

No, but once you see what your checkbook looks like you may want to keep recording until you are sure you are back in balance!

Carbs

Carbohydrates are not the "Bad Guy"

I can't start the conversation about carbohydrates without talking first about the sun. Contrary to all the "low-carb" and "no-carb" diet hype that still cycle through the media, the physiological fact remains your body needs carbohydrates. So why do I mention the sun and carbohydrate together? Let me try to explain in this chapter and perhaps shed some light at the same time on why carbohydrates should not be looked at as the "bad guy". Let's reserve that deserved distinction for high fructose corn syrup or it's aliases corn syrup, corn sugar, HFCS and all the fake sugar substitutes which I'll cover in this chapter too!

To explain the term carbohydrate, start with the sun. Sunlight strikes a leaf and through a complex process — not yet completely understood — the energy in the sunlight is used by chlorophyll (the green coloring matter in the leaf) to manufacture carbohydrate out of the carbon dioxide in the air and water taken up from the soil. This is called *photosynthesis*.

Carbohydrates are the most abundant organic substances. Carbohydrate makes up the <u>structural parts</u> of plants in the form of cellulose as well as stores of starches and sugars.

Carbohydrates are complex molecules composed of Carbon, Hydrogen and Oxygen. One gram of carbohydrate yields 4 kilocalories (or calories) of energy.

The science and importance of mother nature's greens

During daylight hours, green leaves take up carbon dioxide from the air (put there when we breathe). At night the leaves produce oxygen as well as sugars and starches plus cellulose matter that helps the plants stand up and grow larger.

Without this process throughout the plant kingdom, there would be no natural sugars and starches. We would have to obtain energy from protein or fat. You'll understand, as you learn more about nutrition, that all life-preserving processes and substances cannot survive without each other.

- Protein is needed to grow new tissue.
- Fat provides fat-soluble vitamins and protection as well as energy. So the cycle goes. All processes and portions serve one another.
- Carbohydrates provide about half the caloric energy intake for most Americans.

Beware of Low-Carb Diets

Many people think, or are convinced to believe, that to lose weight they must reduce carbohydrate intake. They cut down on bread, cereals and sugars, etc. The truth is, there are B Complex vitamins in grains and cereals and other nutrients. Note: I am not talking about the glow in the dark sweetened kids cereals here, but rather the whole grain non-GMO varieties you can learn about in the resources section.

Reduced carbohydrates presents another complication. If you cut down on carbohydrates and, thus calories, you'll lose weight, but, you'll also "shrink." This is because tissue will not be repaired and replaced properly. Only when the body has enough carbohydrate will it allow protein to build new tissue. When carbohydrate intake is reduced, some of the protein is converted to provide energy.

As a result, tissue loses its ability to repair and rebuild properly. It's dangerous to tamper with one nutrient because it affects many others at the same time.

A Recurring Theme: BALANCE!

A recurring theme in this book and your personalized program is "balance."

There is a balance in the human system that must be maintained. It varies for different people. And that balance also is "governed" by certain endocrine glands such as the thyroid and adrenal glands. Deprive your body of a given nutrient — too often and too long — and the balance becomes disturbed. In addition, other glands and processes in the body begin to strain in an attempt to keep-up their normal duties while trying to compensate for the missing nutrient.

Carbohydrates are broken down and transformed into simple sugars. Some of the glucose (blood-sugar), is used as fuel by the brain, nervous system and muscles. A small portion of glucose is converted to glycogen (a different form of glucose) and stored in the liver and muscles. The excess is converted into fat and stored throughout the body as a reserve source of energy.

"But, What About My Snacks?"

Carbohydrate snacks that contain large amounts of refined sugars and starches promote a sudden rise in blood sugar levels. Thus, they provide the body with an immediate source of energy. The "insulin spike" that follows rapidly lowers the blood sugar levels. This results in cravings for more sugary foods. The end result usually is fatigue, dizziness, nervousness and headaches. Be sure to read the section on high fructose corn syrup at the end of this chapter!

Over indulgence in starches and sweet foods may suppress the desire for other essential nutrients. Often this results in nutritional deficiencies, obesity and tooth decay. Diets that are high in refined carbohydrates are usually low in vitamins, minerals and cellulose.

"I'll Eat Enriched Bread"

Foods such as white flour, white sugar and polished rice are lacking in the B vitamins and other nutrients. Excessive consumption of these foods will perpetuate already existing vitamin B deficiency conditions.

Enriched products usually include some of the B vitamins. If the B vitamins are absent, however, carbohydrate digestion cannot take place, resulting in indigestion, symptoms of heartburn and nausea. Individual variations including rate of metabolism, activity level, body weight and body consumption will significantly influence the total amount of carbohydrates necessary for an individual to function at an optimal level.

Did you know? *A lack of carbohydrates may promote ketosis, loss of energy, depression and the breakdown of lean body tissue.*

Digestion of Starch

The digestion of starch in carbohydrates begins in the mouth and then continues in the small intestine. As mentioned earlier, the main product of carbohydrate metabolism is glucose, or blood-sugar. In this form it enters our blood stream and first supplies the energy needs of our central nervous system. Any glucose not used immediately is stored in the liver or muscles as glycogen. The excess is converted to fat and stored throughout the body. Glycogen reserves are important because this is the primary fuel of hard working muscles and supply of it is limited.

The body can store only a limited supply of glycogen: approximately 350 grams when the supply is at its peak. One-third of the amount is stored in the liver and the remainder in the muscles. Liver glycogen is available for immediate use. It is quickly converted into glucose when needed by the body. Muscle glycogen, however, does not have the necessary enzymes for this direct secretion into body fuel. It furnishes glucose indirectly.

The reserve of glycogen lasts 2-15 hours, depending on activity levels. Someone sitting down and watching T.V. can have enough to last most of the day. Athletes in serious training can use their entire supply of glycogen within 2-3 hours. The body will then switch to alternate, but, less efficient energy fuels. Muscle protein, for instance, can be converted by the liver into glucose in order to keep the brain and nerves supplied with fuel. However, this puts unnecessary stress on the liver. It also drains the supply of amino acids needed for building muscle and repairing the body.

Greens and Fresh Fruits and Vegetables are Best

For healthy weight-management, fruits and vegetables are the best type of carbohydrates and perhaps at the top of that list would be greens!

These natural carbohydrates with long chain sugars and fiber are ideal for replenishing your body with the energy required to fuel your brain, nervous system and muscles.

Remember, refined carbohydrates, like sugar, are so concentrated that they overload the system. The body is equipped to store only limited amounts for energy needs. Cakes, pie, candy, and soda cause the blood sugar to rise. Your body responds by producing insulin, a hormone causing a rapid drop in the blood sugar level. This leads us to a discussion of high fructose corn syrup (HFCS) and the rise in obesity shortly after it was introduced into our food supply. Read on to learn more about Sugar Bombs and the real "bad guys" in the next section.

Don't Skip Carbs
Carbohydrates provide needed fiber, vitamins and minerals in your diet and they are essential for good colon health. Most Americans get less than 10g of fiber daily when for optimal health we should be consuming a minimum of 35g and upwards of 50+g may be best!

Low Carb Debate

My Grade on Low-Carb-Diets

Low carbohydrate, or low-carb-diets are still in fashion for their reported ability to help control blood sugar, and assist with weight loss, blood pressure control, and blood cholesterol control. You may be aware of or have tried several popular low-carb diets, such as the Atkins, South Beach, and Zone diet. When total carbs are reduced, people eat larger proportions of protein and fat. Some low-carb diets recommend replacing carbohydrate with healthful sources of protein and fat; others, such as the Atkins-Diet, do not restrict any type of protein or fat sources. You may find that generally eating fewer carbs may be beneficial, without having to follow a specific program. Recent research demonstrated that after years tracking these popular low carb diets, that they were no better for long term success for weight loss when compared to lowering calories alone.

- The standard diet generally referenced by dietitians provides 2,000 calories, with about 60% of these coming from carbohydrates, which means about 300 grams of carbohydrate per day. Anything less than this could be considered a low-carbohydrate diet. Popular low-carb diets range from almost zero carbs to about 35% (about 175 grams per day).
- Dieters are cautioned against eating less than the Recommended Dietary Allowance of 130 grams of carbohydrates per day (26% of calories in a standard diet).
- Keep in mind that your personal requirements might be more or less than 2,000 calories and I've provided an exchange list to help you plan for a

balanced selection of macronutrients that best meets your own needs.

Take a low-carb-diet for a test drive:

Read nutrition labels on packaged foods to help count your carbs for the day and see where your diet rates for carbs using the guidelines mentioned above. If you'd like to use an online meal planner you can try many free online to help determine if you are following a low-carb-diet. The carbohydrates you choose should be high in fiber such as whole grains, fruits, and vegetables. More of your calories should come from lean meats, fish, beans, low-fat dairy products, and unsaturated, non-hydrogenated oils. I do not recommend this type of meal plan long term especially if you are trying to support exercise and I will explain more at the end of this chapter.

Why do people follow low carb diets?

Many people expect to have better success with weight loss and control of blood pressure, blood sugar, and blood cholesterol levels by following a low-carb-diet. Some specific low-carb-diet programs still being recycled, such as the Atkins-Diet, restrict carbohydrate to the point that the body breaks down fats into ketones, which can either be used either as energy or eliminated from the body via the breath or urine. Diets such as the South Beach and the Zone diets are less restrictive, and some, such as Sugar Busters, seek to eliminate only sugars and high-glycemic-index foods that excessively raise blood sugar.

David Dansereau

The new low carb "danger" diets

The new diet debate which has emerged in the last few years advocates avoiding carbohydrates and all their cousins for their supposed negative effect on both brain and gastrointestinal health. The successful diet books *Grain Brain* by Dr David Perlmutter and *Wheat Belly* by Dr. William Davis both hold carbohydrates as villians. In his diet book, Perlmutter says carbs destroy your brain and he places a good chunk of the blame for the rising tide of Alzheimer's firmly on the dietary recommendations of the past 40 years to eat whole grains. Davis, on the other hand takes a related spin on a term we know so well 'beer belly' with his book *'Wheat Belly'*. Wheat is the central piece of his book as he believes the wheat we eat today bears little resemblance to the wheat our ancestors ate due to genetic engineering. One of the central themes of his book is that gluten intolerance is not just about celiac disease. He believes there is a range of gluten intolerances with celiac disease being at the top of it and modern wheat, bred for more and more gluten is a major challenge for our systems.

Both authors make no distinction of portion control, and perhaps instead should be educating that too much of any one thing is a bad thing. That's why I partly agree and disagree with both of their positions on nutrition and health. To be clear, I don't believe eliminating any one macronutrient is the solution to our Nation's ills and escalating nutrition debt. In fact, we went down that road in the 80's with eliminating fat and replacing it with carbohydrates and now we simply have a situation of portion distortion with carbohydrates! Balance is the key missing ingredient in both these popular diet books, along with the simple fact that they are also both selling supplement and product solutions as part of each of their own branded diet "fixes". Dr. Perlmutter offers a full line of supplements and Dr. Davis pushes his own line of prepackaged gluten free products and other substitutes (which have not been non-GMO verified according to his website). No wonder there is so much diet confusion. With more and more "best selling" solutions like this no wonder many well intentioned readers are drowning in *brain drain* trying to make sense of it all!

I do believe there is a connection with the evolution of wheat and our deteriorating health but I believe this is only a small part of where it all started. Few people know of Norman Borlaug, a University of Minnesota trained geneticist who won the 1970 Nobel Peace Prize for his work in developing a high-yield dwarf wheat that could produce ten times the output of original wheat of its day. At the time, I don't believe it was his intention to cause an epidemic of obesity, diabetes, or Alzheimer's disease. His intentions were to try to feed the world better, prevent starvation and I am sure to improve profits and yield per acre. I believe the significance to the dwarf wheat discovery was that it lead to more advanced genetic engineering (GE) techniques, like the transgenic varieties of seed over the past twenty year that have been pushed on our plates by agribusiness giants without adequate testing. You can read more about this in my included chapter on GMO Nation to learn about all of the food products that are currently produced with GE technologies.

What do the advocates of low-carb say?

Advocates contend that the high amount of carbohydrates in typical modern diets is unnatural for humans, who evolved for hundreds of thousands of years while eating a low-carb-diet. They say that the current over consumption of carbs has led to increasing problems with obesity, diabetes, and other health problems. High-carbohydrate diets are presumed to result in higher insulin levels, which may lead to insulin resistance and related metabolic disorders such as high triglycerides, low HDL ("good") cholesterol, and high blood pressure. Some scientific authorities do recommend that people with the insulin resistance syndrome (IRS) or type 2 diabetes avoid high-carbohydrate diets, and some recommend a diet lower in carbohydrate than current public health guidelines suggest.

Researchers have demonstrated that replacing carbohydrate in the diet with either fat or protein lowers blood triglycerides and raises HDL ("good") cholesterol, and a few studies have also reported improved blood sugar control and increased loss of weight and body fat resulting from these dietary changes.

What do the critics say?

Many nutrition experts disagree with the basic premise of low-carb-diets on the notion that high-carbohydrate, low-fat diets cause obesity and other health problems. In one argument, some nutritionists point to the traditional Japanese diet that is very high in carbohydrates, low in protein, and very low in fat, yet is associated with good health and normal weight in people who follow that diet. Rather than attributing obesity and other problems to carbohydrate intake, these critics blame the overconsumption of calories (from any source) and lack of physical activity as the primary causes of these health disorders. This is the portion distortion concept I mentioned earlier in this chapter.

Critics concede that low-carb-dieters often experience significant weight loss during the initial stages of the diet. However, these critics argue that these diets often have a diuretic effect (in other words, they promote water loss) and that the initial weight loss is due to water loss, not fat loss. Recent research suggests that some people may lose more weight over the course of several months on a low-carbohydrate diet than on one that is equal in calories but higher in carbohydrates, but few studies have been done to determine the long-term effects, good or bad, of low-carbohydrate diets.

In addition, many authorities are concerned that a lower-carbohydrate diet may result in higher calorie intake from fat, which could lead to more difficulties with overweight, insulin resistance, high cholesterol levels, and heart disease risk. Studies of low-carbohydrate diets that are also low in calories and promote weight loss often do not support these concerns, but research on the effects of higher calorie versions of these diets is scarce and conflicting. Increased protein intake as a result of avoiding carbohydrates is also a concern for some critics, since some high-protein diets may increase the risk of osteoporosis, kidney stones, and some cancers.

Critics also express concern that the lack of grains, fruits, and vegetables in low-carbohydrate diets may lead to deficiencies of key nutrients, including fiber, vitamin C, folic acid, and several minerals.

Best food choices on a Low-Carb-Diet

The human body works best with a diet that includes some carbohydrate. Recently a Recommended Dietary Allowance for carbohydrate was set at a minimum of 130 grams per day. This would represent 26% of the calories in a 2,000-calorie-per-day diet, which would still be considered a low-carbohydrate diet, but would avoid the potential hazards of more restrictive diets, including symptoms of ketosis (nausea, weakness, dehydration, light-headedness, and irritability) and loss of body

protein. (See the charts with meal exchanges in this chapter for more help).
Certain dietary fats and their food sources are associated with good health and reduction of disease risks. Foods high in unsaturated fats that are free of *trans* fatty acids have been associated with protection from atherosclerosis, heart disease, insulin resistance, and other health concerns. Examples of these foods include olive oil, fatty fish, flaxseeds, and nuts. However, replacing high-carbohydrate foods with these foods may increase calorie intake if portion sizes are not kept moderate.

Certain sources of dietary protein are more healthful than others. Protein foods containing significant amounts of saturated fat and cholesterol have been associated with many diseases, including heart attacks, type 2 diabetes, insulin resistance, and gallstones; choosing low-fat and low-saturated-fat protein foods can minimize these risks. High meat intake, even of leaner cuts, may increase risk of osteoporosis and kidney stones. Well-done meat or meat that has been preserved with nitrites should be avoided, or kept to a minimum, due to links with cancer. The most healthful choices for increasing protein intake are fish and seafood, small amounts of organic dairy products, legumes, nuts, and seeds.

Even a low-carbohydrate diet should emphasize healthful carbohydrate sources. Whole grains, fruits, and vegetables supply fiber and many important micronutrients. People with diabetes or insulin resistance may find that choosing carbohydrate foods with a low-glycemic index improves their blood sugar, blood cholesterol, and triglycerides; helps them better control their weight; and improves symptoms associated with their health conditions.

Bread, cereal, rice, and pasta
- Whole wheat and whole grain breads
- Breads containing whole, intact grains and seeds (millet, flaxseed, etc)
- Whole wheat pasta and noodles
- Brown rice, basmati rice
- Barley, buckwheat
- Whole grain cereals, muesli
- Whole wheat pita, whole grain wraps
- Steel Cut Oats

Dairy products and dairy substitutes
- Nonfat organic milk and milk products
- Unsweetened organic nonfat yogurt
- Coconut and Almond Milks (unsweetened)

Fats and oils
- Extra virgin olive oil
- Flaxseed oil, hemp oil, pumpkin seed oil, safflower oil, sesame oil, sunflower oil, coconut oil

Protein (meat, poultry, fish, eggs, nuts, and beans)
- Organic lean chicken and turkey
- Egg whites
- Seafood and fish
- Dried beans and peas
- Nuts and seeds

Do low-carb-diets make the grade?

My opinion regarding low-carb-diets:
Many dieters that are also exercising while following a low-carb-diet may find that this meal plan may not provide enough energy to fuel their muscles and support their activity level. I also share the same concerns as other nutrition critics of low-carb-diets that this type of diet may be restricting valuable vitamins and minerals and not providing complete balanced nutrition.

Suggestion: Create a well-balanced weight loss plan that controls calories every day, includes exercise, and allows a wide variety of healthy foods. To lose weight, it is simply not enough to restrict just one type of macronutrient without addressing eating habits that cause weight gain. Take a look at our review of Mediterranean diets for a diet that gets better grades or try our PTC MAP system to help you plan better for success.

Sugar Bombs and the "Fakers"

The Real "Bad Guys" that are giving Carbs a Bad Rap

First, the top villian -HFCS: What is it?

Table sugar is a combination of fructose and glucose which are both simple sugars produced naturally by plants. The combination is called sucrose. Corn syrup is mainly glucose produced from corn starch. There is no naturally occurring fructose in corn which is why fresh uncooked corn isn't sweet. But, in the 1950's, scientists found a way to convert the glucose in corn into fructose. The resulting concoction is 90% fructose (and therefore very, very sweet). That fructose is mixed with the corn syrup, which is glucose (and not sweet), until a 45/55 balance is reached (fructose being the higher percentage). And, presto, HFCS! Later, in the 1970's, the process was scaled and we saw the birth of the HFCS boom.

Coincidental Trend or Damning Evidence?

Once HFCS was introduced in the late 1970s, a cheaper form of sweetener than plain sugar became widely available. It is true that obesity rates have risen by more than 100% since then. The rise in diabetes since 1980 equaled the increase in HFCS consumption according to a study in the American Journal of Clinical Nutrition. There have been various studies conducted comparing HFCS and table sugar. One was a 10 week study that showed after the 10 weeks the HFCS participants had new fat cells surrounding their organs. The table sugar participants showed no new fat cells around their organs.

We now know that HFCS is not good for us and can lead to weight gain and even obesity. There are plenty of studies that show regular sugar can do the same thing and can tip the energy balance scales towards fat gain. But does one type of sugar cause it to happen faster than the other? These studies appear to show that, but in the end they are both just as guilty in contributing to weight gain and obesity.

What to Do?

Instead how about just eliminating or minimizing HFCS and excess table sugar all together. Minimize your processed foods and look at the labels for the words HFCS, corn syrup, corn sugar* and even sugar especially if it is the first ingredient used for that food. There are of course many other unhealthy ingredients that can contribute to your weight gain and perhaps alter your hormone balance and gut flora but I would put HCFS on your short list of ingredients to keep out of your kitchen.

Beware of the marketing hucksters "spin"

*Corn sugar-The "New" "Corn Sugar" is really only High Fructose Corn Syrup (HFCS) in disguise. Yes, it is part of another food industry cover up to help keep marketing this cheap fattening ingredient in the wake of all the negative media surrounding HFCS. The Corn Refiners Association recently petitioned for this name change (HFCS changed to the new corn sugar name) thinking that it would avoid confusion about high fructose corn syrup. Their argument is that HFCS is the same as table sugar.

Bottom Line: Forget about the fake white stuff! If you need something sweet, go for natural foods like real fruit or a small amount of pure local honey as a condiment, or use your blender and make a smoothie using the natural sweetness from fruits.

Fake Sugars

Nutrasweet, Equal, Spoonful, Equal Measure and the new ones in the pipeline are all made with aspartame. Aspartame accounts for over 75% of the adverse reactions to food additives reported to the FDA. I won't even give this topic more than one paragraph. All I can say is this is an ingredient that is foreign to your gut and is connected with way too many adverse effects and diseases to mention. Despite the clear warnings, it remains on the market. Do some research on your own and you'll find the way aspartame was discovered was by accident and later it was delayed and introduced to the market. There were and still are concerns for very real health and safety issues related to the long term use of aspartame products. The manufacturers will deny these claims of course as they aim to keep pumping them into your mouth and gut. Read about the warnings for aspartame on your own but my advice is plain and simple-remove these fake sugars from your diet right away!

Here's a Full List of Excess Sugar and other Sugar Bombs to Avoid:

Sugar and artificial sweeteners. Sugar in agave nectar, barley malt, beet sugar, blackstrap molasses (use sparingly), brown sugar, buttered syrup, cane juice crystals, cane sugar, caramel, carob syrup, castor sugar, confectioner's sugar, corn sweeteners, corn syrup, corn syrup solids, d-mannose, date sugar, demerara sugar, dextrin, dextrose, diastatic malt, diatase, ethyl maltol, evaporated cane juice, fructose, fruit juice, fruit juice concentrate, galactose, glucose, glucose solids, golden sugar, golden syrup, grape sugar, high fructose corn syrup HFCS, honey, icing sugar, invert sugar, lactose, malt syrup, maltodextrin, maltose, maple syrup, molasses, muscovado sugar, panocha, raw sugar, refiner's syrup, rice syrup, sorbitol, sorghum syrup, sucrose, sugar, syrup, treacle, turbinado sugar, yellow sugar. Artificial sweeteners including diet sodas, other artificially sweetened foods, sweeteners including acesulfame potassium, alitame, aspartame, aspartame-acesulfame salt, cyclamate, NutraSweet, saccharin, Splenda, sucralose.

Fats

Infamous Fat – Also Known as Lipids...

Lipids include fats, oils and fat-like substances that have a *greasy* feel. Oil, lard, hydrogenated shortening, butter, margarine, bacon and salad dressings are the most concentrated sources of fat. In fact, as far as energy yield, fats provide the most concentrated energy of all the macronutrients at 9 kilocalories (calories) per gram.

Did you know that FAT can be invisible...?

That's right! "Invisible fat" represents about three-fifths of the total fats you consume. These sources include meats, poultry, fish, dairy products (excluding butter), eggs and baked products.

All of the fat in an egg is in the yolk. Whole milk, cream, ice-cream and whole milk-cheese have appreciable amounts of fats.

Meanwhile, fruit, vegetables, legumes, cereals and flours are very low in fat. Nuts, on the other hand, have an appreciable amount of concentrated fat in the nut oil.

Classified Fat

Fats can be divided and identified as:

- Simple lipids: known as triglycerides which are esters of fatty acids and glycerol. Waxes (or wax like substances) are also esters of fatty acids and long-chain or cyclic alcohols. This group includes the esters of cholesterol, Vitamin A and Vitamin D.

- Compound lipids: including phospholipids such as lecithin, cephalins and sphingomyelin.
- Derived lipids: including phospholipids such as glycerolize, sterols, carotenoids and the fat-soluble vitamins A, D, E and K.

Fat Is a Great Source of Energy

One of the many complexities about lipids is that they digest slowly in the body. Thus, if you eat a meal heavy in fats, they stay in the stomach longer and you feel "full."

Eat too much and you start a nice collection of fat in the liver, metabolic system and in various storage points around your body. (Usually these storage places are where you don't want fat to be stored). Fat also is a rapid source of energy — but only if you work at it.

What Else You Should Know About Fat

There are two dominant forms of fat in the body known as the "Cis" and the "Trans form." Food and body-fats exist principally in the "Cis" forms. This is an important point although a little mysterious. In the manufacture of vegetable shortenings and margarine, some, but not all, of the oil bonds are hydrogenated. They are thus changed from their origin – "Cis form" to a "trans form." Both forms are utilized in the body. But, the Cis form may be better utilized.

Hydrogenation also reduces the linoleic acid content of the fat. These changes have significance in digestion and are believed to affect the rate and manner in which fat is accepted and used in the body. The body does only one of two things with fats. It either stores fat or converts fat to energy.

Fat Storage

This storage problem is not just about large midriffs, flabby arms and enlarged buttocks. The liver is a prime place where the body literally "hoards" fat. It's as though the liver wants to have enough fat just in case energy doesn't come along in the next meal.

Fatty liver is a very serious problem. Among the several fatty substances stored in the liver is one we are familiar with, called cholesterol. This can create problems in the liver if too much is stored. It also is a potential problem if it's released into the blood stream. Cholesterol must keep moving. If it doesn't, it will begin to "cake" or "coat" the interior walls of the blood vessels. It will create obstructions by making the inner diameter of the blood vessel smaller and more narrow.

When referring to fat, a key word to remember is lipotropic. This literally means "to move the fat." There are certain lipotropic substances that <u>must</u> be present and available to prevent accumulation of fat in the liver. They include Choline, Vitamin B-12, Betaine and possibly Inositol.

Through the years, the amount of fats consumed by Americans, day after day, has increased. Less and less do we eat cereals, breads and potatoes. More and more we eat ice cream, fast foods, table spreads as well as other fats. This has created considerable concern in nutritional research. Research shows that a high intake of saturated fats and cholesterol elevates the amount of lipids in the blood. While one watches this steady increase of fatty substances in the blood the world also watches a steady increase in cardiovascular disease.

"How Much Fat is Enough?"

As you progress on your personalized program keep in mind that certain fat soluble vitamins essential to human health are carried in fats. When you reduce fat intake you reduce the intake of these vitamins.

Vegetable fats, such as corn, safflower, and soybean oils, are high in linoleic acid. Nutritionists suggest that Americans should derive no more than 20 to 30 percent of their total daily caloric intake from fats.

Where Fat Comes From?

Meats – All meats contain fat. The percentage of fat will depend on the cut of meat and the grade of the meat. Prime and choice cuts of meat will contain a higher level of fat, which makes them more tender. The standard and good grades are the lower grades. They lack the tenderness associated with the high fat levels and are lower in fat. Not all fowl is low in fat. Duck and goose have a relatively high level. The lowest fat meats are fish, turkey and chicken in that order.

Dairy Products – All dairy products contain fat and cholesterol. However, current studies show that it is healthier to consume the "natural" products over most of the artificially produced dairy products. The heat processing of products that contain fats tends to produce a harmful fatty substance called a "trans-acid." It is best, however, to purchase dairy products that are "low-fat" or "non-fat."

Cooking Oils – There is a large variety of cooking oils sold in the United States. Since most are polyunsaturated they do not raise cholesterol levels nor assist the body in making cholesterol.

Solid Shortenings – Many now have a process that allows them to have a higher percentage of polyunsaturated fat than saturated fat.

Fruits and Vegetables – Most contain some fat but in very low concentrations. Avocados are an exception and are higher in saturated fat than any other vegetable.

Nuts – Most nuts are moderately high in fat content. Walnuts contain the highest levels of polyunsaturated fats while macadamias are one of the highest overall fat nut. Some of the nuts such as cashews and coconut have more saturated fat than polyunsaturated.

More on Omega 3's

Add fat to lose fat?

Yes, if you learn to read the label and add essential fats to your diet that are the correct type. Here's some tips to build your nutrition skillpower and learn how to incorporate healthy fats:

Fats 101

The omega-3 family of fats includes alpha-linolenic acid (ALA), found only in plant foods and considered an "essential" fatty acid because the body cannot make it. Besides flaxseed and walnuts, other sources include canola oil, soybeans, soybean oil and leafy greens like mustard greens.

Two longer-chain omega-3 fatty acids, eicosapentaenoic acid (EPA) and docosahexaenoic acid (DHA), are found in seafood. Fish produce EPA from the ALA in the algae they ingest and then produce DHA from the EPA. Humans can convert ALA to EPA and DHA also, but not nearly as efficiently as fish (and chickens) do.

The Research on Omega 3's

If past headlines didn't motivate you to eat more salmon and sardines for heart health, the latest news on omega-3 fatty acids oils is hard to ignore. Several major studies now attest to the heart-protective power of the omega-3 fatty acids in fish. For the first time, benefits were also found in women as well as men.

Body in Balance

In a study reported in the *Journal of the American Medical Association,* diet information was collected from nearly 85,000 healthy women as part of the ongoing Nurses' Health Study.

"Compared to women who ate fish less than once a month, those who ate two to four servings a week were 31% less likely to develop heart disease over 16 years. Even women who ate as few as one to three servings a month lowered their disease risk by 21%".

Don't like fish?

Here's How to Optimize Plant Sources of Omega-3 Fats

Can you get enough omega-3 fatty acids by eating walnuts and flaxseed?

That can be a challenge. Walnuts and ground flaxseed (flax meal) are recommended sources of an essential omega-3 fat, but if they are your sole omega-3 sources, it's unlikely you'll generate enough of the longer-chain fats that provide many of the health benefits attributed to omega-3's.

Even in healthy people under optimal conditions, scientists estimate that humans have the ability to convert only about 5% to 10% of ALA in walnuts, flaxseed, oils and greens to EPA (and only half of that ultimately converts to DHA). Eating a diet high in trans fats and polyunsaturated fats may further inhibit the conversion.

Benefits of Omega 3's.

Most experts agree that Americans could benefit from more of all three omega-3 fats. EPA has been linked to numerous health benefits, including less risk of blood clots, reduced triglyceride levels and lower blood pressure, thus helping prevent heart attack and stroke. DHA is important for brain development and eye health and for preventing abnormal heart rhythms. And research is now beginning to find that ALA has some impressive health effects of its own. Population studies show that the people whose diets contain the most ALA are at least risk of heart disease.

To get ALA, I suggest eating a small handful of walnuts or adding a tablespoon of ground flaxseed to your cereal (or pancake batter) each day. But to get appreciable amounts of EPA and DHA, you simply can't beat seafood, particularly fatty fish like salmon and sardines.

<u>Take Action:</u> Aim for two+ servings a week of wild caught fish. Supplements can fill in to provide help here but be careful as quality varies considerably. I suggest you use an independent testing agency like Consumerlab.com to see if the fish oil supplement you may be considering has passed testing. I have included a link to the fish oil I use in the resource links for this guide and I will be doing an upcoming webinar on this topic in my Smart Moves Webinar Series.

Protein
Breaking Down Protein

Here's the technical explanation of protein: Protein is the "group name" to designate the principal nitrogen constituents of the protoplasm of all plant and animal tissues. If you listen to the media hype, protein has also become a marketers dream solution to curing all that wrongs you. The truth is we are a sicker, fatter and more tired nation than ever before in history and the reality is eating more protein will not provide a cure. So, with that said, let's discuss why protein is important.

<u>Primary Function:</u> Proteins are necessary for tissue syntheses and regulation of certain bodily functions. Protein provides the same energy return per gram as carbohydrates, with 4 kilocalories (calories) per gram.

However, to say that proteins are more important than other nutrients is not appropriate. An inadequate dietary supply or interference of any nutrient in the body can have serious consequences. Proteins are complex structures made up of amino acids. The type of amino acids vary with each protein. However, nitrogen is always present. Nitrogen in fact is one component that protein has different from carbohydrates and fats in that they do NOT contain nitrogen.

Availability Of Protein

Most menu plans, generally, are well supplied with animal (meat) proteins and amino acids are in generous quantity. But, many conditions can alter the amounts and availability of individual amino acids.

Illness, stress, extreme cooking procedure, etc. all affect foods before they are eaten. On average, most people are good eaters of proteins. However, this does not take into account the very young – who may not be able to eat enough protein or, – senior citizens who may not be able to purchase enough protein due to costs.

All foods provide different amounts, types and combinations of amino acids. An everyday meal plan of meat, milk and eggs will provide a high yield of essential amino acids. But, is this really practical? How many people simply don't like eating meat, milk and eggs every day? And can most people really afford meat, milk and eggs every single day? Meat is, by far, one of the most expensive single items at the grocery store.

Other Sources of Protein

In cereals, millets and similar grains, Lysine and Threonine are the "limiting" amino acids. This means they exist in smaller quantities and NOT in proper balance. For example, corn is deficient in Tryptophan. Legume products are deficient in sulfur amino acids and Tryptophan. Nuts and oil seeds as well as soybean proteins are poor in Methionine. Sunflower seeds lack Lysine.

Peanut proteins (supposed to be one of the most complete foods) are deficient in Lysine, Methionine and Threonine. Green peas are a poor source of Methionine. Green leafy vegetables are a good source of proteins except for Methionine.

The "Official" View

Many of the "official" public health experts like to say, *"It doesn't really matter."* They claim that if you eat a balanced diet of everything — you'll probably get enough amino acids somewhere in that meal plan.

But, the experts are usually talking about the average sedentary individual — not a person embarking on an exercise program with personal individual habits, pocketbooks, likes and dislikes. Therefore, it is reasonable to suggest that individuals with active lifestyles may have amino acid deficiencies that are difficult to identify.

Limiting Amino Acids

The term "essential" refers to a specific nutrient that the body is not capable of producing, but does require. If the essential nutrient is not supplied through diet or supplementation, a deficiency for that particular nutrient may occur.

As with protein synthesis, if one amino acid is supplied in a smaller amount than necessary (i.e., incomplete proteins or low-quality protein), then, the total amount of protein that can be synthesized from other amino acids will be limited. When this occurs, body protein synthesis is restricted. If one essential amino acid is completely absent, however, the other amino acids can not be utilized and are therefore, wasted by the body.

It's All or Nothing

The human body works on the "all or nothing" principle in protein synthesis. Only complete proteins, as opposed to partial proteins, can be utilized. The same situation can occur when an essential amino acid is destroyed as the result of heating protein to extreme temperatures. In this case, all of the other amino acids in the protein become limited. This is referred to as the "limiting factor" of a protein. For example, cooking egg whites may result in a limited protein.

"What if I'm a Vegetarian?"

For years, researchers concluded that vegetarians could easily become protein deficient unless each meal provided a balance of amino acids. Current studies continue to indicate that the body must receive sufficient amounts of the essential amino acids in order to sustain life.

It is now known that protein requirements in vegetarian diets can safely be obtained through a combination of complimentary plant proteins that work synergistically to produce the necessary amino acid balance.

There is much confusion and discussion throughout the research world about supplements of protein and amino acids. The final judge, however, is <u>you</u>. When you gain the results you wish from a protein or amino acid supplement — no amount of authoritative research writing is going to change your mind. Once again, if you do choose to supplement, I would suggest you use an independent lab to verify your protein quality. There has be quite a bit of negative literature lately about high levels of toxic lead and metals being sourced from China and showing up in popular protein supplement brands. Visit Consumerlab.com to subscribe to their reviews. Consumerlab does charge an annual fee to access their site but the information is well worth it.

The scoop on "Paleo"

Paleo Diet: The push to eat like "Cavemen"

What our hunter-gatherer forebears may have eaten in the Paleolithic era (a.k.a. the Stone Age) allowed them to survive and be energized to constantly be on the move as they worked hard for each meal. Things began to take an unfortunate turn (about 10,000 years ago) with the advent of agriculture, more modern tools and the domestication of animals. Now, fast forward to today and our ultra-modern, packaged fast food industry. The only hunting going today is by food lobbyists working for mega-agricultural giants as they track down and dine policy makers in Washington. With the current level of obesity and illness around us, perhaps evolution (and political greed) has been too good to us.

One of the theories behind the Paleo diet is our bodies haven't evolved fast enough to properly handle "new foods" such as grains, legumes, and dairy, let alone the additive-packed processed foods that fill supermarket shelves, so the key to optimal health, according to proponents of paleo is to return to a diet that is closer to that of our distant ancestors.

In a nutshell, that is the underlying premise of the Paleo Diet, which had its beginnings in *The Stone Age Diet*, written by gastroenterologist Walter Voegtlin and published in 1975. Overshadowed by regimens such as Atkins, South Beach, and Meat Lover's, it didn't really take off until a few years ago, with the publication of the bestselling *Paleo Diet* books by Dr. Loren Cordain. Although his website asserts he is "the world's foremost authority on the evolutionary basis of diet and disease," Dr. Cordain's doctoral degree was actually in exercise physiology, not in medicine, the study of the Paleolithic era, or evolutionary biology. Still, the Paleo movement has caught on and unless you're living in a cave (sorry), you've undoubtedly read about or encountered various Paleo diet advocates everywhere you turn. Part of that is we like to be part of "what's new" and we are always up for trying the next best thing, so I wanted to comment here on what I like and don't about Paleo.

What I Like about Paleo

Eating plenty of fresh produce and lean meats and eliminating processed foods from your diet makes perfect sense and is a good thing, no wonder Paleos lose unwanted pounds, and feel invigorated when they make the switch from the very sad, standard American diet (SAD).

What I Don't Like

Cutting out entire food groups such as whole grains, legumes, and dairy because our bodies stopped adapting 10,000 years ago? Not sure that is really how evolution works but then again I simply like chickpeas in my salads too much to go full blown Paleo! I also can't see myself hungry for a raw slab of beef like hard core practitioners do by going full-on caveman (they only eat raw meat!).

Did you know? Insects are a well-documented Paleolithic source of food that modern-day Paleos conveniently ignore!

If you'd like to watch a great video on debunking some of the practices of the Paleo Diet from an archaeologist point of view then follow the link in the resources section for this chapter.

Vitamins and Minerals

Vitamins

The body, itself, produces many substances which may, ultimately, form a vitamin. However, generally, vitamins cannot be made inside the body. Instead they must come from the foods we eat.

Unsolved Mysteries...

These substances, although tiny in amounts, are quite potent and essential for several bodily functions and processes. Some vitamins are soluble in water and others in oils.

Many mysteries still exist about vitamins. Research to identify and isolate vitamins continues in laboratories all over the world. Sometimes they are "discovered" when a human or animal is steadily deprived of certain kinds of foods. The resulting conditions help researchers decide that a specific substance is causing the undesired effect. In other cases, a given malfunction or disorder in the body corrects itself when sufficient amounts of a specific substance is supplied.

"Do Vitamins Supply Energy?"

Vitamins are not "true foods." That is, they don't supply energy, nor do they turn into tissue as do proteins. They do not work like fats or carbohydrates. They have been compared to a catalyst or *spark plug*. They are necessary to make the process work properly or optimally.

As nutritional research moves forward, it is gradually being discovered that a certain vitamin, or combination of vitamins, is essential for health. This is because vitamins combine with enzymes. Vitamins are often termed "co-enzymes."

Simply stated, vitamins are substances that regulate a variety of everyday biological functions in your body. The quantity of each that is needed varies with each vitamin.

Vitamins are essential for normal growth, good health and general day-to-day maintenance.

How to Identify a Vitamin

Two characteristics mark a particular compound for identification as a vitamin:

1. The compound must be a vital organic dietary substance and not a carbohydrate, protein, fat or mineral. It must be necessary in small quantities and perform a specific metabolic function or be useful in preventing a deficiency disease.

2. It can not be produced by the body. Instead, it must be supplied in food. (Vitamin D is the only exception to this rule.)

Vitamin Classifications

Vitamins are classified in relation to their solubility in either fat or water. The fat-soluble group includes Vitamins A, D, E, & K. These vitamins are usually associated with certain fatty foods, such as animal meats, oil or dairy products. These vitamins are more heat-stable than water vitamins. Therefore, less damage occurs during food preparation.

Fat Soluble Vitamins

Vitamin A

There are two basic forms of Vitamin A – performed and provitamin A. The performed vitamin A is found only in animal sources. It is usually associated with fats. The more common provitamin A (carotene) is found in plants. It was first discovered in carrots, thus deriving its name. The majority of human needs are obtained from plant sources, and carotene is converted into usable vitamin A by our bodies. When vitamin A enters your body, certain fat-related substances assist in its absorption. These substances are bile salts, pancreatic lipase and fat itself. The most important functions are in the area of vision and tissue growth. Recent studies, however, associate vitamin A to open-wound healing, severe burn healing, sexual functioning, diabetes, and as a possible aid in treating cancer patients. Sources of vitamin A include colored fruits and vegetables, dairy products, eggs, margarine, fish liver oils and liver.

Vitamin D

Vitamin D also requires the presence of bile salts to assist in its absorption. After being absorbed, vitamin D is carried to the liver and other organs to be utilized. Since Vitamin D is stored in the liver, there may be the same potential for toxicity as in Vitamin A. Vitamin D in the body is concerned mainly with the absorption of calcium and phosphorus. It makes the cell membrane more permeable to calcium and phosphorus, thus allowing the cell to utilize these materials. In the absence of Vitamin D, bones do not form properly, which can cause deformities during a child's growth years. Vitamin D has other key roles in the body, including modulation of cell growth, neuromuscular and immune function, and reduction of inflammation. Vitamin D can be produced endogenously (inside the body) when ultraviolet rays from sunlight strike the skin and trigger vitamin D synthesis. Food sources of Vitamin D in nature are somewhat limited. These include the flesh of fatty fish (such as salmon, tuna, and mackerel) and fish liver oils which are among the best sources. Small amounts of vitamin D are found in beef liver, cheese, and egg yolks. Many packaged cereals and milk products are often fortified with vitamin D.

Vitamin E

Vitamin E has been found to be a group of related vitamins. It is fairly stable to heat and acids, but can be destroyed by alkaline. One of the most important characteristics is its ability as an anti-oxidant. Vitamin E may be found in eight different tocopherol forms. However, most products contain only the alphatocopherol, and most contain the synthetic form. The synthetic form can be differentiated from the natural form by the appearance of a small "1" after the "d"?(i.e.:, d1-alpha tocopherol = synthetic). Food sources of Vitamin E are mainly vegetable oils. Other food sources include: milk, eggs, wheat germ, fish, green leafy vegetables, and cereals.

Vitamin K

Vitamin K has been known as the blood clotting vitamin. The major function of this vitamin is to control the synthesis of prothrombin. Prothrombin, which is produced by the liver, is necessary to initiate the blood clotting process of the body. Vitamin K is normally synthesized by the bacteria in the intestinal tract. An adequate supply is normally present in the average healthy person. The use of antibiotics, however, may destroy or reduce the effectiveness of the intestinal bacteria in producing adequate supplies. It is therefore suggested that when on antibiotic therapy, substances that provide material to rebuild bacteria (such as acidophilus) should be considered. The first Vitamin K was derived from alfalfa which is still a good food source. Other sources include: green leafy vegetables and small amounts from cheeses, tomatoes, and liver.

Water Soluble Vitamins

B Vitamins

B Vitamins are directly related to three main areas of our nutritional needs and support system. The first group includes: thiamin, riboflavin, and niacin, which relate to alleviating various disease factors. The second group includes pyridoxine and Pantothenic acid which have a role in providing coenzyme factors to the body. The third group includes folic acid and B12 which are important blood-forming factors.

Vitamin B1

(Thiamine) The absorption of Thiamine takes place mostly in the first section of the small intestines, the duodenum. Removal of either part or all of the duodenum resulting from an ulcer or injury will significantly affect Vitamin B absorption due to its being destroyed by alkaline intestinal secretions found in the lower intestinal tract. Thiamine is not stored in large quantities in the body. Therefore, daily intake is important. Its main metabolic function in our bodies is as a coenzyme in key reactions that produce energy from glucose. Clinical effects that may relate to a B1 deficiency may be seen in the gastrointestinal, nervous and cardiovascular systems

Vitamin B2

(Riboflavin): Absorption of B2 takes place mainly in the upper section of the small intestines. Similar to B1, B2 is a vital factor in protein metabolism and is also a part of a key enzyme system relating to the production of energy in the cell. B2 deficiencies rarely occur alone. They are usually associated with other nutritional deficiencies. The best source of B2 is milk. Other sources include: organ meats, whole grains and some vegetables.

Vitamin B3

Niacin (Nicotinic Acid): Niacin teams up with riboflavin as a control agent in the cell coenzyme system that converts protein to glucose. Deficiencies of niacin are closely related to those of riboflavin. They may include: weakness, loss of appetite, indigestion and skin eruptions. Niacin also has a close relationship to Tryptophan. When Tryptophan is present in adequate amounts, a niacin deficiency will _not_ occur. Our body utilizes the Tryptophan to produce the niacin.

Vitamin B5

(Pantothenic Acid): Pantothenic Acid is widespread throughout the body. It is synthesized in considerable amounts by intestinal bacteria. Because of this, production deficiencies are unlikely. Pantothenic Acid assists in cellular energy production. It also is essential for the formation of acetylcholine (the regulator of nerve tissue) and assists in the production of cholesterol, steroid hormones and Vitamin D. Some sources of Pantothenic acid are: yeast, liver, egg yolk and skimmed milk.

Vitamin B6

(Pyridoxine): B6 is absorbed in the upper portions of the small intestines and is usually found throughout the body tissue. B6 is essential in deamination and transamination which involve moving nitrogen around to form different amino acids.

Vitamin B9

(Folic Acid): The absorption of folic acid takes place throughout the small intestines. Small amounts may be synthesized by intestinal bacteria. A deficiency of folic acid produces a nutritional megaloblastic anemia. This large blood cell is unable totransport oxygen properly.

Vitamin B12

(Cobalamin): Vitamin B12 was discovered during the search for a specific agent to control pernicious anemia. B12 is unique and one of the most complex of the B vitamins. Its uniqueness comes from its chemical makeup which reveals the mineral cobalt at its core. B12 is the only human nutrient known that requires exposure to HCL in the stomach before it can be absorbed. The HCL prepares the vitamin and allows it to be absorbed. Improper absorption of Vitamin B12 is the key factor in pernicious anemia. Sources of B12 are almost solely animal foods. The best sources are liver and dairy products.

Biotin

Biotin is a coenzyme necessary for a variety of important functions in our bodies. Biotin helps in the metabolism of carbohydrates, proteins and fats. It is needed for normal growth, healthier hair and skin and maintenance of nerves, bone marrow, and? sex glands. Sources are yeast, liver, eggs, whole grains, and fish.

Choline Bitartrate

Choline Bitartrate has a relationship to fat metabolism. If the body has a problem breaking down fat, the fats have a tendency to be deposited in the tissues of organs, such as the kidneys, liver, heart and vascular system. Excessive quantities of fat in these organs interfere with the normal functioning of the cells and may be a cause of premature aging of that organ.

PABA

PABA (Para-amino benzoic acid): This is a member of the B-complex family. It stimulates intestinal bacteria to produce folic acid, and is involved in the utilization by the body of Pantothenic acid. PABA is most widely known as a good therapeutic sunscreen.

Inositol

Inositol is a member of the B-complex family. It occurs in high concentrations in the brain. Inositol may have a cholesterol-lowering quality. It has a tendency to break up fat in our systems when given with Choline.

Vitamin C

Vitamin C is absorbed from the small intestines. It is not stored or produced by the body. Therefore, an ample supply must be taken in daily. It is a very unstable vitamin and can be destroyed by oxygen, alkalines, high temperatures and light. Since it's easily destroyed, cooking vegetables and fruits should be kept to a minimum. Also the more surface of a vegetable that is exposed to air, the less Vitamin C content will be retained. Vitamin C acts as an intercellular cementing substance. It also helps to build and maintain bone and connective tissue. It aids information of hemoglobin, is active in wound healing; helps fight infections; maintains body resistance against a variety of ailments and maintains strong blood vessels. Sources include: Citrus fruits, vegetables, potatoes, strawberries, green pepper, broccoli, melons, etc.

Minerals

Minerals are an essential group of nutrients that act in the body as control agents. They are significant in energy production, cell reproduction and body maintenance.

The role that minerals play in our metabolism is varied, yet, vital. Minerals are essential for structuring iron's relationship to the blood cells, cobalt's relationship to B12 as well as sodium and potassium controlling body fluids.

Minerals are categorized into two groups: The major minerals which are present in large amounts and trace minerals which are present in smaller amounts.

Major Minerals

Calcium

Calcium is present in the human body in the largest amount. An adult of approximately 150 lbs. has three pounds of calcium in his or her body. The quantity of calcium consumed and amount that is actually utilized by the body varies depending on a number of factors controlling absorption and utilization.

Physiological functions of calcium:

- Bone and teeth formation
- Blood clotting
- Helps contract and relax muscles
- Normal nerve impulse transmission
- Cell wall permeability — regulates fluid passage
- Helps transport nerve impulses
- Major factors in regulation of heart muscle.

Food sources of calcium are: dairy products, green leafy vegetables, nuts, and whole grains.

Phosphorus

The same factors that control calcium absorption in the body also determine the quantity of phosphorus absorbed. Phosphorus is closely related to calcium in many functions, but is found in the body in a smaller quantity (approximately 1.5 lbs. in a 150 Lb. man).

Physiologic function of Phosphorus:

- Absorption of glucose
- Transport of fat
- Helps maintain pH of blood
- Essential for energy metabolism
- Strong bones and teeth.

Sodium

Sodium is a crucially important mineral. It has numerous metabolic roles in the body. It is a major electrolyte in the extra-cellular fluids and helps regulate the body fluids.

Physiologic functions of sodium:

- Regulates the acid-base balance through a buffer system
- Controls the sodium pump in cell walls, allowing a cell wall to become permeable to potassium and other materials
- Helps transmit electrochemical impulses to help stimulate muscle action
- Deficiency may cause stomach and intestinal gas.

Excessive sodium intake can cause edema (a fluid accumulation). Sodium requirements are normally met by the body from our diet. Added sodium is rarely needed. Sources include: milk, eggs, carrots, leafy green vegetables and a large percentage of processed foods.

Potassium

Potassium – Similar to sodium, potassium is an element associated with water balance. Potassium is approximately twice as plentiful as sodium. The majority is located inside the body cells. Potassium is absorbed from the small intestines and almost all dietary potassium is absorbed.

Major physiologic functions:

- Water and acid-base balance
- Regulates the neuromuscular stimulation; normalizes heart beat
- Aids in CHO metabolism and protein synthesis
- Joins with phosphorus to send oxygen to the brain
- Stimulates kidneys to dispose of body wastes
- A deficiency may cause constipation, insomnia, slow and irregular heart beat

- Diuretic drugs may have a tendency to deplete the body stores of potassium and a supplement may be needed.

Magnesium

Magnesium - Approximately 70% of all magnesium in the body is combined with calcium and phosphorus in the bone. The remaining 30% is in soft tissue and body fluids. It functions as an enzyme activator in energy production and tissue protein synthesis.

Physiologic functions:

- Plays an important role as a coenzyme in the building of protein
- Helps keep you calm and cool – relaxes nervousness
- Deficiency may lead to renal calculi.

Chloride

Chloride – Chloride is a constituent of body fluids outside the cells. It helps control water balance with sodium. It also assists in acid-base balance.

Sulfur

Sulfur – Sulfur is an essential constituent of cell protein. It also is an active component in energy metabolism.

Trace Minerals

Iron

Iron plays a vital role in our bodies, especially in the area of blood-building and energy production. The body levels are controlled by the dietary amounts consumed and the amounts in the liver that are constantly being used in the production of hemoglobin. Iron is absorbed by the intestines with the aid of special cells which receive the iron and transport them in the body.

Factors affecting the absorption of iron:

- Body demands
- Vitamin C aids by helping to change dietary iron to a usable form
- HCL (hydrochloric acid) helps prepare iron for absorption
- Adequate calcium as binding agent and to remove phosphate which hampers absorption.

Physiologic functions:

- Hemoglobin formation. Hemoglobin is the oxygen transport carrier
- Helps convert glucose to produce energy
- Deficiency may cause a variety of animias
- Iron-weak persons may have poor memory due to brain being starved for oxygen.

Iodine

Associated mainly with the thyroid gland, only a small amount is needed. The body's needs are adequately supplied by the use of iodized salt. It is absorbed in the small intestines and transported around the body with the assistance of proteins. Approximately one-third of all iodine absorbed is utilized by the thyroid gland, the balance being excreted in the urine.

Physiologic functions of iodine:

- Synthesis of thyroid hormone
- Deficiency causes slow mental reactions
- Needed to utilize fat
- Shortage may cause rapid pulse, tremors, nervousness, increased irritation.

Fluorine

There is not a single process in your body that requires fluoride. Fluorination is a chemical process where a fluorine atom in integrated into a molecule. When you hear about fluoride in drinking water, it comes from adding a fluorine compound (usually sodium fluoride) to drinking water. There are over 100 published studies illustrating fluoride's harm to your brain. Even advocates that say fluoride has some role in the prevention of dental decay still warn there are dangers with overexposure. Consider that too much fluoride could be ingested with what is added to drinking water and being overexposed to this mineral daily with every food item you consume or prepare that had been made with unfiltered "tap" water. There is also controversy in the literature on both sides of this debate. I would contact your water supply board in your local area and ask for their water quality report which will indicate if fluoride is added to the municipal supply as well as any violations the department may have been cited for. You should know that Brita, Pur and most other home filters do not remove fluoride. Reverse Osmosis Filtration does remove fluoride but these systems are mostly not affordable for personal use.

Lithium

Very successful at one time in treating manic-depressives and other mental illnesses. May have a role in prevention of Alzheimer's Disease

Copper

Copper is essential for hemoglobin synthesis, probably by promoting the absorption, mobilization and utilization of iron.

Manganese

- Works with B-complex vitamins to overcome sterility
- Combines with phosphotase (an enzyme) to build strong bones
- Can biologically substitute for iron in heme molecule
- Is deficient in chronic alcoholism
- Promotes lactation

Selenium

Selenium can substitute for Vitamin E in certain animal species. Selenium is a natural antioxidant. It works closely with vitamin E in some of its metabolic actions and in the promotion of normal body growth and fertility.

Zinc

- Constituent of insulin and of male productive fluid
- Combines with phosphorus to aid in respiration
- Helps the food become absorbed through intestinal wall
- Essential to nucleic acid metabolism and protein synthesis

- Deficiency may be a factor in atherosclerosis
- Women who take oral contraceptives are usually zinc deficient.

Molybdenum

- Possible role in iron utilization
- Deficiency may result in renal calculi.

Chromium

Physiologic functions:

- Necessary for normal glucose utilization
- Deficiency may be related to increased incidence of diabetes in later life
- Is usually deficient in pregnancies and malnutrition
- Deficiency may be caused by an excess of white sugar

Cobalt

Physiologic functions:

- Constituent of vitamin B12
- Related to healthy hemoglobin formation.

Boron

Boron is an essential trace mineral believed to be related to vitamin C activity.

The Only Time to Fast

Your Evening Fast is the Only Time to Diet

Quarantine Your Kitchen Close the Kitchen after dinner to starve your fat cells at night!

If there is one lesson I have learned after years of learning about nutrition, studying the human body and behaviors, and working with clients to help them achieve their fitness, diet or rehabilitation goals it is this one very important point. It is rarely on little thing that a person does to sabotage their efforts, whether it be to lose body fat, gain muscle or rehab successfully from an injury. Rather it is a bunch of little things that have an accumulated effect.

Here's a perfect example and I'll use myself to illustrate a point. Not many people know this but I have a nacho problem. Really. I can pass on a party full of sweets-rich chocolate cake, ice cream, cookies-not a problem. However, if I know there are organic (non-GMO) nachos anywhere in the house I'll hunt them down in a weak moment. Especially, if I know their companions are also calling- a real cold Sam Adams and a jar of mildly spicy salsa. Ahhhh-heaven! * My ever loving spouse knows this very well and she does her best to keep nachos off the shopping list unless on the rare occasion we need them for entertaining. Even then, at my request, she sneaks them in the house and tries to keep them clear of the "danger zone"-that being my mouth.

* [**Personal Sidebar**] *That little bit of heaven lasts up until I almost kill the whole bag, then I realize how awful I feel after, but it is too late. Yes, nachos are like a potent drug in my body, and I overdose easily.*

The point of this introduction is that we all have weaknesses, especially when it comes to food. I have counseled hundreds upon hundreds of clients in nutrition and I know all too well that in order to really do well on a plan, you must not have your temptations or food triggers in your pantry.

When I refer to quarantining your kitchen, I am referring to removing all the toxic elements that you know could potentially sabotage your efforts. Take an inventory of all the junk items, convenience snacks, and other processed foods that you know could end up in your mouth and on your hips or behind in a moment of weakness. Also refer to the section on GMO foods and be sure to start the process to remove these items from your shopping list as well.

Clear out the junk now before you even make your list to start your next shopping trip.

As you are throwing out or donating these items take note of all the saturated fat, especially trans fats as well as sodium and simple sugars. Your heart and waistline thank you already.

Action Step: Instead of procrastinating and saying you'll keep the tempting items until they are gone or until someone else finishes them, just remove them. Stop kidding yourself. You'll end up eating them. Please go and complete this action step today!

Kitchen Closed.

When you are trying to lose excess body fat you must do anything except come back to the kitchen for an evening snack right before bed.

Suggestions:

Have water with lemon or apple cider vinegar, enjoy a cup of decaf green tea, go for a walk, have sex, go to sleep early-ANYTHING but FEEDING your body before bedtime. It does not need the food at this time. Anything you consume when your body is shutting down for the evening is readily stored as extra energy supplies -and those little fat cells are always ready to take in energy.

Why?

With late night eating you are actually signaling your body to prepare for more activity, but the mindless eating that usually goes on at this hour is from stress or boredom. Late evening is the other key time of day where even the best designed plans get ruined.

Those extra 200-300 calories at the end of the day will destroy your fat loss efforts every time.

Points to consider: Some of the same chemicals or hormones released during our primitive fight-or-flight stress response are also responsible for gauging the anticipated use of those extra calories we just consumed while watching television. The body does not have a good anticipation meter of calories you might burn sitting vs. telling your body I am fueling now to run a marathon. The end result if you do not go out and burn off those extra calories is that cortisol stimulates fat cells deep in the belly to store that extra energy.

Remember: **Fuel** Your Muscles all Day long –**Starve** Your Fat Cells at Night!

I'll try a "simple shake for breakfast and lunch" and a sensible meal for dinner approach and that should work, right?

Most who use this method end up teaching their bodies how to store fat. There are many reasons for this costly mistake but the answer is based in simple physics. The main diet blunder here is that most folks who try and fail at this approach don't have a clue how to plan a sensible dinner. Instead, they have conditioned their body to eat like a pigeon all day long by sipping on their meals in a can when their bodies actually need real nutrition and energy from food. To make matters worse, they gorge like an elephant in the evening when they should be signaling their body to slow down and prepare for rest.

Canned diets or shakes of any type do not teach skill power. Instead, these "quick-fix" diets or liquid "diet cleansing programs" set off your body's defense mechanism against rapid calorie deprivation with the end result being a slower metabolism and loss of lean muscle.

The other little known dirty secret of the pre-packaged diet food industry is that most companies including the "big ones" you see advertised every year with their flashy New Year's marketing plans can't even follow through with quality ingredients. Here's a short list of some of the companies that are known to use GMO ingredients and other artificial, questionable additives in their shakes and meal replacements:

Shakeology, Herbalife, Jenny Craig, Nutrisystem, Slimfast, Ensure, Atkins, Isogen, Pure protein, Muscle Milk, Shaklee, MonaVie, most of the popular energy bars. See the Non-GMO resource list for shopping for on the go alternatives.

You might want to check with the supplement manufacturers themselves. For example, here's a copy of what Nutrisystem states about what's in their line:

"Nutrisystem makes every effort to provide high quality food products made from the best ingredients. This <u>does include some ingredients that are genetically modified.</u> Please note that foods containing genetically engineered ingredients are subject to controls and regulations by U.S. federal agencies, and must meet the same strict guidelines for food safety as all food products."

You'll find if you do some calling and research of your own most of the packaged foods are cutting corners and using cheap, genetically modified ingredients!

Exchange your Notion of Being on a Diet

Balancing Your Food Choices

Here's a few meal templates using exchanges (servings*) to help plan your calories for the day (once you've established your own RMR) and ensure you are receiving complete balanced nutrition.

Weight Loss / Weight Maintenance
(with traditional Carbohydrate / Calorie Level)

	1000-1200	1200-1500	1500-1800	1800-2000	2000-2200
Fats	2-3	2-3	3	3	4
Dairy	1	1-2	2	2-3	2-3
Protein	5-6	6-7	7-9	8-9	9-10
Veggies	3+	3+	3-4+	4-5+	4-5+
Fruits	2-3	3	3-4	3-4	4-5
Starches	5-6	6-8	8-9	9-10	9-10

Weight Loss / Weight Maintenance
(100-130g Moderate Carbohydrate Calorie Level)

	1000-1200	1200-1500	1500-1800	1800-2000	2000-2200
Fats	2	2-3	3	3-4	4
Dairy	1	1-2	2	3	3
Protein	9-11	11-12	13-16	16-17	17-19
Veggies	4	5	5	5-6	5-6
Fruits	2-3	3	3	3	3
Starches	2	2	3-4	4	4-5

Weight Loss
(35-50g) Very Low Carbohydrate Calorie Level

	1000-1200	1200-1500	1500-1800
Fats	2-3	3-4	4
Dairy	0	0	0-1
Protein	14-15	17-20	20-23
Veggies	3-5	4-5	5
Fruits	1	1	1
Starches	0	0	0

I've provided this very low carbohydrate template mainly to show individuals where calories would have to come from when carbohydrates are eliminated in order to maintain energy. For many, this is an extreme change and unsustainable long term along with perhaps being challenging for to the body to have to deaminate or breakdown all that protein daily. For more help with meal templates consider our PTC Map System which you can learn more about in the resources links.

Another method of looking at how your daily plate could be divided is to visualize your plate accordingly into five categories: (40%)veggies, (20%)lean protein, (20%)healthy fats, (15%)fruits and fiber, and a small dose of (5%)nuts and dairy.

*Exchange List Serving Sizes

Fruits contain 15 grams of carbohydrate and 60 calories.
One serving equals:
- 1 small Apple, banana, orange, nectarine
- 1 med. Fresh peach
- 1 Kiwi
- ½ Grapefruit

- ½ Mango
- 1 C Fresh berries (strawberries, raspberries, or blueberries)
- 1 C Fresh melon cubes
- 1/8th Honeydew melon
- 4 oz Unsweetened juice
- 4 tsp Jelly or jam

Vegetables contain 25 calories and 5 grams of carbohydrate.
One serving equals:
- ½ C   Cooked vegetables (carrots, broccoli, zucchini, cabbage, etc.)
- 1 C   Raw vegetables or salad greens
- ½ C   Vegetable juice

Lean Protein choices have 55 calories and 2–3 grams of fat per serving.
One serving equals:
- 1 oz Chicken—dark meat, skin removed
- 1 oz Turkey—dark meat, skin removed
- 1 oz Salmon, swordfish, herring
- 1 oz Lean beef (flank steak, London broil, tenderloin, roast beef)*
- 1 oz Veal, roast or lean chop
- 1 oz Lamb, roast or lean chop
- 1 oz Pork, tenderloin or fresh ham
- 1 oz Low-fat cheese (with 3 g or less of fat per ounce)
- 1 oz Low-fat luncheon meats (with 3 g or less of fat per ounce)
- ¼ C 4.5% cottage cheese
- 2 med. Sardines

Fats contain 45 calories and 5 grams of fat per serving.

One serving equals:
- 1 tsp Oil (vegetable, corn, canola, olive, etc.)
- 1 tsp Butter
- 1 tsp Mayonnaise
- 1 Tbsp Salad dressing
- 1 Tbsp Cream cheese
- 2 Tbsp Lite cream cheese
- 1/8th Avocado
- 8 large Black olives
- 10 large Stuffed green olives
- 1 slice Bacon

Fat-Free and Very Low-Fat Milk contain 90 calories per serving.
One serving equals:
- 1 C   Milk, fat-free or 1% fat
- ¾ C   Yogurt, plain nonfat or low-fat
- 1 C   Yogurt, artificially sweetened

Starches contain 15 grams of carbohydrate and 80 calories per serving.
One serving equals:
- 1 slice Bread (white, pumpernickel, whole wheat, rye)
- 2 slices Reduced-calorie or "lite" bread
- ¼ (1 oz) Bagel (varies)
- ½ English muffin
- ½ Hamburger bun
- ¾ C Cold cereal
- 1/3 C Rice, brown or white, cooked
- 1/3 C Barley or couscous, cooked
- 1/3 C Legumes (dried beans, peas or lentils), cooked
- ½ C Pasta, cooked
- ½ C Bulgar, cooked
- ½ C Corn, sweet potato, or green peas

- 3 oz Baked sweet or white potato
- ¾ oz Pretzels
- 3 C Popcorn, hot air popped or microwave

Take note of the portion sizes here for especially for starches. Most individuals have trouble understanding what is in a serving, especially for starches. In most restaurants for example the typical serving of pasta on an American plate is 5-6 cups or more –which is 10x the single suggested serving of ½ cup! With this example, you can see how "portion distortion" is certainly playing a role in giving carbs and starches a bad reputation!

Add Greens - Remove GMOs

The Power of Greens and the Problem with GMOs

[WARNING] If you listen to only one piece of advice from this guide, make it this chapter on what to include and what to exclude from your diet to best begin eating clean!

Remove GMOs-What You Need to Know

What is a GMO?

A GMO (genetically modified organism) is the result of a laboratory process where genes from the DNA of one species are extracted and artificially forced into the genes of an unrelated plant or animal. The foreign genes may come from bacteria, viruses, insects, animals or even humans. Because this involves the transfer of genes, GMOs are also known as "transgenic" organisms.

This process may be called either Genetic Engineering (GE) or Genetic Modification (GM); they are one and the same. There is growing concern and controversy about the safety of GM foods and little scientific proof they are safe for human consumption. Meanwhile manufacturers and the big argri=business giants are working hard with paid lobbyists to protect their profits and spending millions in every state in the US with lawsuits to make sure you don't have the right to know what is in your food. Learn more in the chapter at the end of this guide on GMO Nation to learn how to stay clear of GMO foods. The more you know, the better you'll be able to maneuver around the poisons on your plate, and consequently, the better you'll feel. I know from years of working with clients that making this one simple change to their diets (eliminating GMOs) made profound improvements to their health, even before they adopted healthy exercise habits!

Why Add Greens?

Greens are the closest thing humans have to injecting pure high octane fuel into our cells to generate power to promote blood building nourishment.
Here's why:
Although all fruits and veggies of color have great health properties, the green group occupies the top part of the food spectrum for color because they are the most alkaline of all foods and contain the highest nutrient density. Greens also provide the richest source of chlorophyl, the pigment that gives plants their green color and captures energy from the sun (see the chapter on carbohydrates to learn more about where all human energy begins!).

Did you know? *Only about one-quarter of American adults eat three or more servings of vegetables a day. If you are in the majority who does not, you are missing out on major benefits, as consuming fresh vegetables is one of the key cornerstones to optimal health!*

There is little that compares to the nutritional value of organic, raw vegetables, and according to new research, eating your greens may be even more important than previously imagined.

The Importance of Eating Your Greens

Researchers at Walter and Eliza Hall Institute's Molecular Immunology division (Australia's oldest medical research institute) have discovered that a gene, called *T-bet*, which is essential for producing critical immune cells in your gut, responds to the food you eat—specifically leafy green vegetables. According to their press release:

"The immune cells, named innate lymphoid cells (ILCs), are found in the lining of the digestive system and protect the body from 'bad' bacteria in the intestine.

They are also believed to play an important role in controlling food allergies, inflammatory diseases and obesity, and may even prevent the development of bowel cancers.

... [T]he research team revealed T-bet was essential for generating a subset of ILCs which is a newly discovered cell type that protects the body against infections entering through the digestive system.

'In this study, we discovered that T-bet is the key gene that instructs precursor cells to develop into ILCs, which it does in response to signals in the food we eat and to bacteria in the gut,' Dr Belz said. 'ILCs are essential for immune surveillance of the digestive system and this is the first time that we have identified a gene responsible for the production of ILCs.'"

ILCs are thought to be essential for:

- Maintaining balance between tolerance, immunity and inflammation in your body
- Producing interleukin-22 (IL-22), a hormone that can protect your body from pathogenic bacteria
- Maintaining healthy intestinal balance by promoting growth of beneficial bacteria and healing small wounds and abrasions in the gut
- Helping resolve cancerous lesions

More Reasons to Eat Your Veggies

Vegetables contain an array of antioxidants and other disease-fighting compounds that are very difficult to get anywhere else. Plant chemicals called phytochemicals can reduce inflammation and eliminate carcinogens, while others regulate the rate at which your cells reproduce, get rid of old cells and maintain DNA. So when I told you at the beginning of the guide you have the DNA to be healthy, you just need to feed it, I meant it! To learn more about each phytochemical color see the chapter on food and inflammation.

Studies have shown that people with higher vegetable intake have:

- Lower risks of stroke, type 2 diabetes, high blood pressure, Alzheimer's disease and heart disease
- Lower risks of certain types of cancer, eye diseases and digestive problems
- Reduced risk of kidney stones and bone loss
- Higher scores on cognitive tests
- Lower biomarkers for oxidative stress
- Higher antioxidant levels

Further, if you eat your veggies raw, you'll also be receiving <u>biophotons</u>, the smallest physical units of light, which are stored in, and used by all biological organisms -- including your body. Vital sun energy finds its way into your cells via the live food you eat, in the form of these biophotons. They contain important bio-information, which controls complex vital processes in your body. The biophotons have the power to order and regulate, and, in doing so, to elevate the organism -- in this case, your physical body -- to a higher oscillation or order.

Generally, the more sunlight a food is able to store, the more nutritious it is. Think this is crazy? If you are into computers you know that the first computer was literally built with a lightbulb and these punch-cards which had holes in them. This "old school code" was and continues to be how we program computers. Today the modern silicon chip is used to relay "0's and 1's" but they are interpreted as "<u>lights</u> on, <u>lights</u> off."

Boost Your Body's Computer

Now our sciences are revealing humans work the same way as computers where light carries information through our brain, nervous system, and even our DNA. How do we power our bodies? Naturally-grown fresh vegetables, raw sprouts, and sun-ripened fruits are rich in light energy. Ideally, look for fresh, non-GMO produce that is organically grown on a local farm in your area. Choose the vegetables that appear freshest first, and consume them raw shortly after purchase for optimal benefits.

If you can't obtain organic, conventionally-grown vegetables are better than none! Just take extra care with non-organic vegetables by washing them thoroughly and removing peels and cores when possible to minimize your exposure to pesticides. Certain fruits and vegetables also tend to be far more contaminated than others simply because they're more susceptible to various infestations and therefore sprayed more heavily. Some foods are also more "absorbent," with thin, tender skins. Such foods would be high on your list for buying organic. These foods have earned the name "dirty dozen" because of their higher probability of having the highest pesticide load used to get them to market.

David Dansereau

Here are the "dirty dozen"

(try to buy these organic):

- Apples
- Strawberries
- Grapes
- Celery
- Peaches
- Spinach
- Sweet bell peppers
- Nectarines (imported)
- Cucumbers
- Cherry tomatoes
- Snap peas (imported)
- Potatoes

Plus these which may contain organophosphate insecticides, which EWG* characterizes as "highly toxic" and of special concern:

- Hot peppers and Blueberries (domestic)

In addition, the Environmental Working Group (EWG) produces an annual shopper's guide to pesticides in produce that you can download. It lists the produce with the highest and lowest levels of pesticide residue, which can help save you money if you can't afford to buy everything organic.

From their latest report here were the cleanest produce, or the produce which had the lowest pesticide load. Nearly all of the data used took into account how people typically wash and prepare produce - for example, apples were washed and bananas peeled before testing. Of the fruit and vegetable categories tested, the following "Clean 15" foods had the lowest pesticide load, and consequently are the safest conventionally grown crops to consume from the standpoint of pesticide contamination:

Here are the "Clean 15"

- Avocados
- Sweet corn
- Pineapples
- Cabbage
- Sweet peas (frozen)
- Onions
- Asparagus
- Mangoes
- Papayas
- Kiwi
- Eggplant
- Grapefruit
- Cantaloupe (domestic)
- Cauliflower
- Sweet potatoes

How to Quickly Boost Your Greens
Try some of my smoothie recipes to get started going green! More smart smoothies recipes are online in the resources.

Smart Moves Greenie
4 cups kale, swiss chard, or dark lettuce
1 apple
1 frozen banana
1 pear (or 1/c cup of pineapple)
Juice of 1 lime (or lemon)
2 tsp chia or flax seeds
2 tablespoons of walnuts, almonds or hemp seeds
½ cup water

David Dansereau

Smart Brain Blast
2 cups of spring greens
1 cup blueberries
1 avocado
1/4 cup walnuts or pumpkin seeds
1/2 cup blackberries
1 frozen banana
2 tsp chia or flax seeds
1/8 cup fresh ginger shavings
1/2 cup unsweetened coconut milk or water

Case Studies: Bodies Back in Balance

Sharing a Few Client Stories
(with their permission of course)

"Rachel" became the inspiration for the first edition of this book.

"A client of mine I'll refer to as Rachel, was in the process of selling her home and expanding her business simultaneously. She was an artist and the practice of making her craft involved very physical demands. She originally came to me because she felt exhausted and she was developing aches and pains, especially over her neck, shoulders and low back. She was also a recreational rower, having previously skulled competitively in college. After a comprehensive physical evaluation, we developed an eating plan and exercise routine to match the demands she was placing on her body. Our goal in this plan was not to add additional stress, but to incorporate focused movement and eating strategies that would rebalance and refuel her muscles with the intention of making her daily activity simpler.

After the chaos of her business expansion had settled down and she got "refocused" Rachel found great reward in the exercise regimen we had developed. She reported that she was no longer overstressed and by completing our periodic fitness re-evaluations together we determined she had added valuable muscle tissue and reduced fat. She was thrilled as her body fat level had decreased from 24% at our initial evaluation to 18% in a period of 6 months. Rachel ended up eventually selling her home and moving out of state to merge her growing business with a partner and I didn't see her again for over 3 years. I incorrectly assumed that the tools and lessons she had learned while with me would be enough to help keep her moving in the right direction and on a safe maintenance program. Turns out I was wrong.

I ran into her at a business conference this past summer and her posture, her demeanor, and her walk indicated that she was no longer enjoying the exercise benefits. She confessed that she stopped working out altogether because "the routine stopped working." I was baffled by her comment and at first, I admit now that I took it personally. (A routine that I had designed stopped working?) Then she went on to explain that after she moved away to her new location, she could not find someone to work with her. She explained that she enjoyed having someone to help her establish new goals and monitor her success. It turns out my services provided the motivation she needed to keep moving and a tool for her to stay challenged. That was the answer, the routine didn't stop working . . . it just became a very manageable workload and was no longer challenging. Her body did not have to continue to change as it had developed sufficiently to handle the rigors of the routine. Rather than abandoning exercise, had Rachel recognized that all she needed were a few modifications in her routine, she could have continued a process of continuous and ongoing improvement. It turns out that this mindset of Rachel's would have a profound effect on me and as a result, there is some good news to this story. After our accidental meeting, I was inspired to somehow help Rachel to re-commit and get moving again and I knew I had the tools even with the distance that now was between us. It was then I realized I had not been putting it to use in my practice. To change this, I quietly began making the time to complete a project I had been working on for more years than I care to mention. (Let's just say designing this tool began back in the day when a slender Oprah took the stage pulling a wagon full of "fat" to demonstrate how much weight she had lost on a liquid diet, and then resumed again around the time a Susan Powder was proclaiming that we should all "stop the insanity".- Remember her?)

[Personal sidebar] Wow, I have been at this health and wellness thing a long time!

I digress, what I did was I used this chance meeting with Rachel to make the time and finally commit to completing a revised edition of this crazy guidebook concept that I had been working on for all these years. Turns out that with some extensive tweaking and updating for the computer age, the ideas in my original guidebook which may have been at first ahead of their time were in fact worth the wait. You see, now many of the helpful links and tools in my digital edition and through QR codes in the print edition can be at your fingertips when back during the original draft I actually had question marks next to key points where it meant to me –"how can I make this happen?" Anyway, I want to thank Rachel and the more than a dozen other clients since her that provided a great focus group to test and refine these ideas. It has been by their combined efforts and feedback since my initial meeting with Rachel that I have ultimately been able to add even more valuable content and resources to the now ever expanding Smart Moves Guidebook series.

The end result with Rachel:

She finally found the right balance, employing the same principles you are reading in this book. She did this by starting back with a variation of the routine she was accustomed to (which now was a "new stimulus" since he'd abandoned it for a significant period of time) and over time I restructured or updated Rachel's program by (remotely) using some of the VIP coaching resources I have available   in the resource section of the guidebook. For example, by reducing the time between her exercise movements, modifying the set and rep schemes, and adding in some new exercise combinations all at the correct intervals we perfected a plan to help her reach her goals. Rachel used the Smart Movement screen and resources available in this guide to know just when it was time to update her routine, before it became routine. The real exciting part to this story is that Rachel lives almost 800 miles away and she's enjoying the same success she had when she was a regular client of mine!   Rachel also uses some additional tools I now have available online including my weight management course to help her stay motivated. Today, she is in what she is referring to as the best shape of her life at 46 years old!   It turns out that the same roadblock that Rachel experienced when she first quit because "the routine stopped working" was a similar mindset that I took on years ago when I had abandoned this guidebook project because I was frustrated about my book "not working". In the end, I think we both learned that adapting to a situation, or asking the body to perform slightly beyond that which it's accustomed to is a challenge worth taking. Thanks again "Rachel!".

Memorable Metabolism Makeovers

Metabolism Makeover # 1

The new mom Karen

Karen, age 31, 5'4" 136 lb.

Bodyfat 28% Lean Body Mass 72%

Resting Metabolic Rate (RMR) 1420 calories

Activity Calories Burned: 1060

Average Total Expended: 2480 calories/day

Average Calories consumed: 1800 to 1900

Her Body Goal: Getting back to her pre-pregnancy weight of 130 pounds.

Her Healthy Diet Goal: Cutting out junk food and breaking the "grab something quick" cycle that sabbotages her efforts to eat well. "When my energy gets low I just eat anything that's available" to raise my blood sugar as fast as possible. Then I feel horribly guilty that I ate so poorly when I know better.

Her Fitness Status: Stays active by keeping up with her 22-month-old son who is always "on the move". Karen also fits in a 20 minute treadmill and light weight training routine 2-3 days per week.

Her RMR Test and My Analysis: The one thing that new moms need to remember is their own physical needs, even while they run around taking care of their child's. Karen's diet was analyzed using the food records she provided to me and had entered in using my MAP online activity and meal planner. My analysis revealed she had a fairly well balanced diet and was getting most nutrients in balance except for total calories, calcium, vitamin D and fiber.

Like many of my female clients Karen does not get enough calcium. She also needs to make sure she consumes enough total calories because motherhood is physically demanding. Carrying around a 25- pound baby is serious exercise! While metabolism gets a boost during breast-feeding, thanks to the extra energy it requires to produce milk, your post-motherhood metabolism should not vary significantly from your pre-motherhood one- unless, of course, your weight or body-fat percentages changes dramatically.

Metabolism Makeover:

First of all Karen is doing quite well. She could stay on track nutritionally by setting herself up with quick but healthy meals like 1/2 sandwiches, low sodium soups and mixing in whole grain breakfast cereals with yogurt and fruit. I suggested she have items like these pre-portioned in single serving containers to take "to go". Prep them the night before and be prepared for those situations when low energy times draw you to bad food choices. I also suggested she use the resources on my website to get additional meal templates to print out and have on hand to help provide a guideline for her calorie level.

Finally, I suggested she needed to try to up the tempo of her exercise routine by completing a more intense circuit training cycle 3 non-consecutive days per week. I had her download a copy of my Smart Moves Circuit for home use by going to my exercise membership site. My Smart Moves Circuit is an effective way to boost metabolism by alternating aerobic and muscle building (and metabolism revving) anaerobic moves. For example, fast walk on the treadmill for 6 minutes, then do "baby" squats or lunges for 90 seconds, then plyometric jumps for 30 seconds, biceps curls with shoulder rotational presses to fatigue, then return to the treadmill, etc.

In addition, I suggested she take one day per week to complete a longer walking workout with her son/family. I encouraged her to map out a 30-40 minute safe course in her neighborhood that was not "too flat". Pushing a jog stroller up an incline can be a very effective interval workout. Adding this additional day would also get her outside, away from the treadmill at least one day per week to add to the variety of her routine and spend more time just having fun!

Metabolism Makeover # 2

Tall and "naturally" thin college grad student

Sherri, age 23, 5'9" 127 lb.

Bodyfat 17% Lean Body Mass 83%

Resting Metabolic Rate (RMR) 1240 calories

Activity Calories Burned: 640

Average Total Expended: 1880 calories/day

Average Calories consumed: 2100 to 2400

Her Body Goal: Gain a better awareness of the foods she eats and how that affects her mood and overall energy level.

Her Current Diet: A lot of junk food. Typically a croissant and coffee every morning for breakfast, french fries and diet coke at least 4 times per week by take out. "Most days" include a Krispy Kreme doughnut with a large latte or coffee in the afternoon before sitting down to study. Poor selection of food most days, "only time I see a vegetable" is when I go out to dinner on weekends with my fiance.

Sherri's Fitness Status: She does not exercise presently and would be interested in adding a few more curves to her figure.

Her RMR Test and My Analysis: Sherri's concern about her poor diet and food selection effecting her mood was the main focus of our initial meeting. Even though she was not experiencing problems managing her weight she had requested an RMR measurement because she was sure her metabolism had slowed down "or something" because her energy level was so low.

She reported the daily afternoon coffee and donut were a habit she had developed to keep her awake to get her studies done each afternoon. Her RMR result may be OK now but at such a young age it is important for Sherri to realize that if her bad habits continue after years of not exercising and eating badly, it will eventually catch up to her.

Even though a girl like this who is naturally tall and thin will probably not ever get seriously overweight on Body Mass Index (BMI) charts, she eventually will gain body fat and lose valuable muscle. She is a perfect example of someone who could eventually still rate well by commonly used measures like BMI but actually could almost double her bodyfat as she ages!

Here's how: When's she's 50, let's assume she might even actually weight the same as she does now, but her body composition (ratio of lean to fat body weight) will have definitely changed. After all those years of inactivity she will have lost about 15 pounds of muscle. This will have slowed her metabolism down so much that eating the same amount will have caused her to gain 15 pounds of fat. As a result, her bodyfat will have hiked up from the current 17 percent now to just over 30 percent later.

Also her tall stature and her current avoidance of exercise, especially the lack of any strength training, will put her at increased risk for osteoporosis later in life. I demonstrated to Sherri how her poor nutrition and exercise habits now will make it likely that she would grow frail later in life. I think that visual helped her, even though she certainly didn't come to see me to get a visual of herself in her 50's!

Metabolism Makeover: I know you don't want to hear this but I suggested to Sherri that she probably could get away with a minimal amount of exercise and still make significant improvements in the amount of lean muscle mass she maintains. I discussed with her the important role of cardiovascular fitness and improved endurance capacity for improving her energy levels as well as beginning a meal plan that had some "real foods". When most of your calories are served out of foam containers and brown take-out bags, you are not eating real food. Even though Sherri was not eating an enormous amount of food in total it was certainly all the wrong food and the average total intake for the day was over what she typically was expending. Also when I showed Sherri just how poor her diet rated on my MAP online meal planner, I believe it really opened her eyes how much improvement was needed.

Finally, I also suggested a strength routine that also incorporated a focus on some of Sherri's postural (mid/upper back and core muscles) as she demonstrated the beginning of poor (forward head and shoulder) posture. Her abdominals were also very weak for someone her age. I started her on this mini-workout, my Smart Moves Take Ten routine she could work in as study breaks, several days per week. She later came back to me after 3 months where we advanced her to a full body routine to address some of the muscles she was interested in to "add a few more curves" to her figure.

Note: I have been using metabolic testing successfully in my practice to demonstrate to clients how important understanding this vital sign is to their weight management success. If you have more questions on this topic I have included information about RMR testing in the resources page.

Stress Inflammation and Disease Connection

What is the Root Cause?

Cortisol is a hormone released in response to fear or stress by the adrenal glands as part of the fight-or-flight mechanism. The adrenal glands are endocrine glands that sit on the top of the kidneys.

The fight-or-flight mechanism is part of the general adaptation syndrome defined in 1936 by Canadian biochemist Hans Selye of McGill University in Montreal. He published his revolutionary findings in a simple seventy-four line article in *Nature*, in which he defined two types of "stress":

- eustress (good stress)
- distress (bad stress)

Both eustress and distress release cortisol as part of the general adaption syndrome. Once the alarm to release cortisol has sounded, your body becomes mobilized and ready for action—but there has to be a physical release of fight or flight. Otherwise, cortisol levels build up in the blood which wreaks havoc on your mind and body.

Eustress creates a "seize-the-day" heightened state of arousal, which is invigorating and often linked with a tangible goal. Cortisol returns to normal upon completion of the task. Distress, or free floating anxiety, doesn't provide an outlet for the cortisol and causes the fight-or-flight mechanism to backfire. Ironically, our own biology—which was designed to insure our survival as hunters and gatherers—is sabotaging our bodies and minds in a sedentary digital age. What can we do to defuse this time-bomb and how does it relate to damaging inflammation?

Think about your relatives and friends as case studies

Just like the uncle you may know that already had a heart attack, a great aunt may have two debilitating diseases-rheumatoid arthritis and multiple sclerosis (MS). A close friend may have colitis and their spouse may have asthma. An entire family may have a host of seemingly unrelated ailments like atherosclerosis, chronic obstructive pulmonary disease (COPD), type 1 diabetes, and even depression. All these diseases, despite what you may have been told to "treat" them (with drugs) all have stress and inflammation as the common underlying factor. As scientists are starting to deeply understand the mechanisms of different organ systems, they are also beginning to realize that what occurs in any one system often plays out in another. They are also looking at how possible gene mutations might be effecting the gene "microbiome" (how genes, their microbes and the environment interact). When was the last time your doctor told you to look at your diet as a contributing factor, if not the root cause of your ailment?

Because I already know the answer to the previous question, I will provide you with this information on diet and inflammation to get you started putting out the flame and getting to the root cause of the problem.

Is your heart aflame?

Conventional wisdom at one time in medicine saw heart attacks as caused by a buildup of plaques that eventually blocked blood flow to the heart. A more complicated truth to heart disease and an eventual heart attack is now emerging, one that is showing that the heart is actually aflame, or inflammation has a vital role in the process.

> *" But I thought inflammation was a good thing, and it signaled my body to start to heal from an injury. Is this not true? "*

Inflammation is a key component of the body's healing system; the normal response to injury or irritation. You have most likely known the four cardinal signs of inflammation of swelling, redness, heat, and pain. Inflammation serves to bring more blood and immune activity to an injured area. But it is most important that inflammation stay where it is needed and that it ends when it has served its purpose. Prolonged or inappropriate inflammation becomes a problem and can predispose the body to disease.

Abnormal inflammation is the root of accelerated aging and almost all chronic diseases. Chronic inflammation causes injury to our tissues, specifically the nervous system and gut (where most of out immune complexes reside). Inflammation in the gut allows proteins to leak through the membranes into the blood stream causing inflammatory allergic responses that may influence exacerbations. Inflammation in the brain also causes the ability for toxic substances to cross the blood brain barrier. Other conditions which are the result or worsened by chronic inflammation include Chrohn's/Colitis, multiple sclerosis (MS), arthritis, heart disease, asthma, diabetes and all autoimmune illnesses and obesity.

One theory behind why our immune system becomes inflamed is that our diet has drastically changed from what we ate for thousands of years during the Paleolithic times and our guts have not been able to adapt. Our current over-processed, genetically modified and chemically laden foods are increasingly unfamiliar to our immune systems causing an inflammatory response (allergy-like). Returning to a more natural, less processed whole food diet is more consistent with our genetic make-up and can calm the immune system response thereby reducing inflammation.

Although there are many powerful anti-inflammatory drugs available, such as steroids, or non-steroidal anti-inflammatory drugs, they are not without significant side effects. Fortunately, we can modify inflammation naturally by adjusting our diets. These changes may take 6-8 weeks to notice the results of the diet, but they will occur. I have provided a sample Eating Guide as a subchapter to follow which includes inflammation fighting foods as a bonus for purchasing this book. For now, let's dive a little deeper into stress to see why it is keeping you from losing unwanted bodyfat.

"How Can Stress Affect My Weight?"

It's difficult to avoid stress. Stress enters our lives daily. It can impact your well-being and success on any type of fitness program.

Here is a bit of basic information regarding stress and psychological factors regarding lifestyle changes.

Different Strokes for Different Folks

Stress can mean different things to different people. A roller coaster ride is a thrill to one person — a terrifying experience to the next. Stress is essentially a good or bad change which evokes a generalized physiological response of the body to physical, psychological or environmental demands.

Emotional and physical reactions to stress can become bothersome. Most of us would like to avoid the point where they overflow and disable us. Therefore our bodies have provided a warning system.

Feelings – Feelings are a good signal (anxiety, depression, anger, etc.). Unfortunately, most of us have learned to suppress feelings.

Bodily Reactions – Body reactions are another good warning system to monitor stress including:

- Easily overexcited, irritability, depression
- Increased heart rate
- Dryness of the throat
- Impulsive behavior, emotional instability
- The overpowering urge to cry or run and hide
- Inability to concentrate
- General disorientation, alcohol or drug addiction
- Accident proneness
- Feelings of unreality, general weakness, dizziness
- Fatigue – paranoia
- Body trembling, increased medication use
- High-pitched nervous laughter
- Stuttering
- Grinding of the teeth (bruxism)
- Insomnia, nightmares
- Inability to take a relaxed attitude
- Perspiring
- Frequent urination
- Diarrhea, indigestion

- Neck or lower back pain
- PMS
- Migraine headaches
- Loss of appetite

The Role of Hormones and Nerves

Throughout your body, all processes are precisely and automatically regulated by hormone and nerve activity. It is done so without conscious effort. The central nervous system acts as the control unit. It evaluates all activities both inside and outside your body to monitor and adjust to changing conditions.

The stress response illustrates how the entire body reacts to anything perceived as a threat to your stability or equilibrium.

Both physical and psychological stressors elicit the body's stress response. Major physical stressors include surgery, burns, and infections. Other major physical stressors include, an extreme hot or humid climate, toxic compounds, radiation, and pollution.

Also, chronic "little stresses" or hidden day-to-day issues can lead to *real physical ailments.* Good examples are:

- Family conflicts
- "I hate my job"
- Lack of time, or lack of organization
- Too much responsibility
- No one understands why I'm stressed"
- Rush hour traffic.

And then there are major life changes such as:

- Death or loss of a loved one
- Serious illness or accident

- Divorce or separation
- Death of a close relative
- Getting fired or laid off of work
- Marriage
- Major personal property loss (fire, theft, vandalism)
- New household member.

Stress response begins when your brain perceives a threat to your equilibrium. The sight of a car hurtling toward you; the terror that an enemy is concealed around a nearby corner; the excitement of planning for a party, a move, a wedding; the feeling of pain; a snarled traffic jam or any other such disturbance perceived by the brain serves as an alarm signal.

Alarm Reaction

Once the body perceives stress, it prepares to fight or flee from potentially threatening situations. A chain of events unfolds through nerves and hormones to bring about a state of readiness in every body part. The end result is a preparedness for physical action (fight or flight). Here is a brief description of your body's alarm reaction to stress:

The pupils of your eyes widen so that you can see better. Your muscles tense up so that you can jump, run or struggle with maximum strength. Breathing quickens to bring more oxygen into your lungs and your heart races to rush this oxygen to your muscles so that they can burn the fuel they need for energy.

Your liver pours forth the needed fuels from its stored supply, and fat cells release alternative fuels. Body protein tissues break down to back up the fuel supply and to be ready to heal wounds if necessary. The blood vessels of your muscles expand to feed them better, whereas those of your gastrointestinal tract constrict; and gastrointestinal tract glands shut down (digestion is a low-priority process in time of danger). Less blood flows to your kidney so that fluid is conserved, and less flows to your skin so that blood loss will be minimized at any wound site. More platelets form, to allow your blood to clot faster if need be. Hearing sharpens, and your brain produces local opium-like substances, dulling its sensation of pain, which during an emergency might distract you from taking the needed action. Your hair may even stand on end - a reminder that there was a time when our ancestors had enough hair to bristle, look bigger and frighten off their enemies.

Resistance

This tightly synchronized adaptive reaction to threat is one of the miracles of the human body. You may have performed an amazing feat of strength or speed during an alarm reaction to stress. Anyone can respond in this magnificent fashion to sudden physical stress for a short time.

But if the stress is prolonged and especially if physical action is not a permitted response to the stress, then it can drain the body of its reserves and leave it weakened, worn and susceptible to illness.

Much of the disability imposed by prolonged stress is nutritional; you can't eat, can't digest your food or absorb nutrients, and, so can't store them in reserve for periods of need.

All three energy fuels — carbohydrate, fat and protein — are drawn upon in increased quantities during stress. If the stress requires vigorous physical action and if there is injury, then, all three are used. While the body is busy responding but, not eating, the fuels must be drawn from internal sources. I've provided you with chapters on the macronutrients and vitamins and minerals to help you better understand why each fuel and nutrient in needed in balance to best reduce stress needs.

Stress to Exhaustion

As for other nutrients, they are taken from storage — as long as supplies last. But supplies for some are exhausted within a day. Thereafter, body tissues break down to provide energy and needed nutrients. The body uses not only dispensable supplies (those that are there to be used up, so to speak, like stored fat), but also functional tissue that we don't want to lose, like muscle tissue.

During severe stress, the appetite is suppressed. The blood supply is diverted to the muscles to maximize strength and speed. So, even if food is swallowed, it may not be digested or absorbed efficiently. In a severe upset, the stomach and intestines will even reject solid food. Vomiting, diarrhea or both are these organs' way of disposing of a burden they can't handle. To tell people under severe stress to eat is poor advise. They can't. And, even if they force themselves to eat, they can't assimilate what they've eaten. The same goes for athletes, and this is why timing of meals becomes important with competition.

Stress, Overeating & Fasting

In times of less severe stress, a person may respond by overeating. Many people eat excessively in response to stress since food can have a relaxing effect. The release of some stress hormones often occurs when the body is in need of sugars. You can develop a conditioned response so that whenever stress hormone levels become high, you feel the need to eat. The stress hormone produces insulin resistance, which in turn leads to excess insulin production, fat deposits, and inhibition of fat breakdown.

On the other hand, fasting is itself a stress on the body. The longer a person goes without eating, the harder it is to get started again. So, it can be a no-win situation. It is a downward spiral when people let stress affect them to the point where they can't eat. And, not eating makes it harder for them to handle the stress.

Get a Handle on Stress

It's important not to let stress become so overwhelming that eating becomes impossible. To manage overwhelming stress may be a psychological task, and if too extreme may require the help of a counselor or therapist.

When you can't eat you will lose nutrients. If you can eat under stress do so. Eat more often to meet your nutrition and energy requirements. Supplements can be useful to help prevent the risk of marginal vitamin and nutrient deficiencies, but don't rely on them over whole foods.

Stress has a detrimental effect on muscle, vitamin and nutrients. What measures can we take to minimize them?

The best nutritional preparation for stress is a consistent, balanced and varied menu plan and lifestyle that meets your metabolic requirements. The right nutritional program combined with a regular exercise program will minimize the effects of stress.

Exercise is Stress Relief

One of the best ways to reduce the symptoms of stress is with exercise. Although the causes of stress may be mental, these are physical problems that are curbed with physical activity.

Some factors which may explain the effectiveness of exercise for reducing psychological stress:

- Exercise is a diversion which enables the person to relax due to change in environment or routine.
- Exercise is an outlet to dissipate emotions such as anger, fear, frustration.
- Exercise produces biochemical changes which alter psychological states.

Regular exercise may increase the secretion of endorphins in the brain. Exercise has an effect on your emotional reaction to stress. It does this by altering your mood. Fit people are usually in high spirits after a lengthy exercise (runner's high). This feeling is associated with the presence of endorphins, which are released by the pituitary gland in the brain.

The word endorphin, comes from the combination of two words, Endo and Morphine, meaning endogenously produced morphine. Endorphins are the body's natural pain reliever. It may be the brain interpreting exercise as a form of pain. Or it may be that the rise in fatty acids caused by long, gentle exercise acidifies the blood which triggers release of endorphins.

Stress Therapy

Exercise is what your body wants to do under stress: It burns off some of the stress chemicals that tension produces. Also note that a tired muscle is a relaxed muscle.

Regular exercise reduces anxiety and depression and allows you to cope more effectively with psychological stress. This is effective stress therapy.

Relaxation may be induced through mental exercise as well.

One of the single most important points you can make about stress is that in most cases it's not what's out there that's the problem, it's how you react to it.

Exercise (Breathe!)- Think Positive - and Keep Smiling are the Fasted Stress Busters I know. I go into more details in the chapter on 5 simple strategies to lower stress.

Eat Clean: Foods that Reduce Inflammation

Start with an oil change!

When your car begins to bonk and run poorly, the first thing your mechanic will do is check your service records for your car engine maintenance or look under the hood and be sure you have oil in your engine. Unfortunately, our bodies don't have obvious "check engine" lights but in a way we do. Symptoms such as pain, fatigue, bloating, indigestion, headaches, insomnia, are in fact our bodies way of letting us know attention is needed. Stress and inflammation play perhaps the biggest role in exacerbating all these symptoms so the first thing you should think about doing is check the type of oil your body has been operating on.

The primary steps of the anti-inflammatory diet are as follows:

Reduce refined polyunsaturated vegetable oils (omega-6) (soybean, corn, sunflower, and safflower). We get enough of these naturally in the foods we eat. These oils turn into inflammatory chemicals once metabolized. The goal is to reduce the ratio of Omega-6 to Omega-3 oils to reduce inflammation. Since the American diet has an overabundance of polyunsaturated fats, reducing our intake can help this ratio. It is estimated that the typical American diet has an unhealthy ratio of Omega 6 to Omega 3 of approximately 20:1 when we should be trying for at least a ratio of 6:1 or less (even better a 1:1 ratio). No wonder most American desperately need an oil change!

ELIMINATE ALL TRANS FAT (Partially hydrogenated oil such including margarine, vegetable shortening, and all foods containing trans-fatty acids). These are man-made fats unfamiliar to our immune system and produce inflammatory hormones called prostaglandins (PGE-2).

Reduce saturated fats from animal proteins. Choose small amounts of wild and grass fed meats like we ate in caveman times instead of domesticated grain-fed ones. Also mostly all conventionally fed animals today are fed with GMO grains!

Instead of polyunsaturated oils, rely on monounsaturated, extra-virgin olive oil or unrefined canola oil for cooking and eating. Eat your fat in natural foods like nuts, nut butters, avocado, and seeds or seed oils.

Increase your intake of omega-3 fatty acids by eating wild salmon, mackerel, black cod, high omega-3 eggs, sardines, walnuts, freshly ground flax seeds or oil, greens, and whole soy foods. The omega-3 fats in these foods increase the production of anti-inflammatory hormones called prostaglandins (PGE 1 & 3). You can also take fish oil supplements with DHA & EPA (2-4g/day). Make sure the supplements are free of PCB's and mercury.

Strengthen the immune system with plant foods!

Make sure your diet includes plenty of fresh fruits and vegetables.

Flavonoids in plants protect cells from inflammation. Pick those known for their high antioxidant (cancer preventing) content. Usually, these are the most richly colored and pungent flavored. Eat 6-9 servings or more per day of fruits and veggies. Blue and purple colored plants especially protect the blood brain barrier. So eat your blueberries!

Go For Color in Your Fresh Foods

Here's a quick summary of the foods you should stock up on and a brief summary of why they are so important for disease prevention and blood sugar control. <u>Goal:</u> Try eating at least one serving from each group daily.

How to Color Code Your Kitchen

Color Code: Red

Key Phytonutrients: Lycopene, a carotenoid

Benefits: Induces enzymes that help protect cells against carcinogens; strong antioxidant properties; may protect against prostate and lung cancers.

Best Food Sources: Grapefruit or juice, pink. Pasta sauce, Tomatoes or juice, Tomato soup/sauces/puree, Watermelon

Color Code: Red / Purple

Key Phytonutrients: Anthocyanins, powerful antioxidants

Benefits: Prevent the binding of carcinogens to DNA; may help protect against gastrointestinal cancers.

Best Food Sources: Apple, red, Bell pepper, Blackberries, Blueberries, Cabbage, red, Cherries, Cranberries/ juice,

Eggplant, Grapes or juice, red, purple, Plums, Prunes, Strawberries

Color Code: Orange

Key Phytonutrients: Alpha- and beta-carotene

Benefits: Improve communication between cells, fight the spread of cancer; may help prevent lung cancer.

Best Food Sources: Apricots or nectar, Cantaloupe, Carrots or juice, Mango, Pumpkin, Squash, acorn or winter, Sweet potato

Color Code: Yellow

Key Phytonutrients: Beta-cryptothanxin (a carotenoid)

Benefits: Inhibit cholesterol synthesis needed to activate cancer cell growth.

Best Food Sources: Grapefruit or juice, yellow, Nectarine, Orange or juice, Papaya, Peach or nectar, Pineapple or juice, Tangerine or juice

Color Code: Green

Key Phytonutrients: Sulforaphane, isothiocyanate, indoles

Benefits: Stimulates the release of enzymes that break down cancer causing chemical in the liver; may inhibit early tumor growth

Best Food Sources: Bok Choy, Broccoli, Brussel Sprouts, Cabbage, Cauliflower, Kale, Swiss Chard, Watercress

How Chronic Stress Damages Your Brain

Why Cortisol is Public Enemy #1 to Your Brain

Neuroscientists have discovered how chronic stress and cortisol can damage the brain. A recent study actually reconfirms the importance of maintaining healthy brain structure and connectivity by managing chronic stress.

Neuroscientists at the University of California, Berkeley, have found that chronic stress triggers long-term changes in brain structure and function. Their findings might explain why young people who are exposed to chronic stress early in life are prone to mental problems such as anxiety and mood disorders later in life, as well as learning difficulties.

It has long been established that stress-related illnesses, such as post-traumatic stress disorder (PTSD) trigger changes in brain structure, including differences in the volume of gray matter versus white matter, as well as the and size and connectivity of the amygdala. However, researchers are just beginning to understand exactly how chronic stress creates long-lasting changes in brain structure which affect how the brain functions.

In a series of revolutionary experiments, Daniela Kaufer, UC Berkeley associate professor of integrative biology, and her colleagues, discovered that chronic stress and elevated levels of cortisol can generate more overproduction of myelin-producing cells and fewer neurons than normal.*

David Dansereau

Chronic Stress Changes Neural Networks

The "gray matter" of the brain is densely packed with nerve cell bodies and is responsible for the brain's higher functions, such as thinking, computing, and decision-making. But gray matter is only half of the brain matter inside our heads, the other half of brain volume is called white matter.

White matter is comprised of axons, which create a network of fibers that interconnect neurons and creates a communications network between brain regions. White matter gets its name from the white, fatty myelin sheath that surrounds the axons and speeds the flow of electrical signals between neurons and brain regions.

"We studied only one part of the brain, the hippocampus, but our findings could provide insight into how white matter is changing in conditions such as schizophrenia, autism, depression, suicide, ADHD and PTSD," Kaufer said. The hippocampus regulates memory and emotions, and plays a role in various emotional disorders and has been known to shrink under extended periods of acute stress.

The researchers found that hardening wires, may be at the heart of the hyper-connected circuits associated with prolonged stress. This results in an excess of myelin—and too much white matter—in some areas of the brain. Ideally, the brain likes to trim the fat of excess wiring through neural pruning in order to maintain efficiency and streamlined communication within the brain.

Cortisol Can Trigger Stem Cells to Malfunction

The 'stress hormone' cortisol is believed to create a domino effect that hard-wires pathways between the hippocampus and amygdala in a way that might create a vicious cycle by creating a brain that becomes predisposed to be in a constant state of fight-or-flight.

Chronic stress has the ability to flip a switch in stem cells that turns them into a type of cell that inhibits connections to the prefrontal cortex, which would improve learning and memory, but lays down durable scaffolding linked to anxiety, depression, and post-traumatic stress disorder.

Kaufer's lab focused on neural stem cells in the hippocampus of the brains of adult rats under acute or chronic stress. These stem cells were previously thought to mature only into neurons or a type of glial cell called an astrocyte.

However, the researchers found that chronic stress made stem cells in the hippocampus mature into another type of glial cell called an oligodendrocyte, which produces the myelin that sheaths nerve cells.

The finding suggests a key role for oligodendrocytes in long-term and perhaps permanent changes in the brain that could set the stage for later mental problems. Chronic stress decreases the number of stem cells that mature into neurons and might provide an explanation for how chronic stress also affects learning and memory, according to the researchers.

"Usually the brain doesn't make much oligodendrocytes in adulthood from those neural stem cells," according to Kaufer. In fact, a recent study suggested these cells were incapable of producing oligodendrocytes, which are somewhat like a vine spreading out and wrapping around axons, both insulating and supporting them.

Rats who have high levels of cortisol and chronic stress had fewer neurons overall but a big increase in oligodendrocytes. By blocking the equivalent of cortisol receptors, the researchers discovered the process was tied to the stress hormone.

Although this sheath is vital to human brains—myelin formation can be good or bad, depending on time or place, according to Kaufer. This excessive sheathing may have evolved to bolster the connection between the amygdala and hippocampus, which would improve fight-or-flight responses during extended periods of threat or attack... Unfortunately, in a modern world, chronic stress can hijack the fight-or-flight system and backfire in a daily life in which you are not in physical danger.

Conclusion: Plasticity Makes it Possible to "Sculpt" Your Brain Throughout a Lifespan

Regular physical activity and mindfulness meditation are two effective ways to reduce stress and lower cortisol. Although this study doesn't focus on the benefits of reducing cortisol, other research suggests that making lifestyle choices that reduce stress and lower cortisol can improve brain structure and connectivity.

For a simple way to lower cortisol without drugs check out the chapter in this book on types yoga and breathing techniques.

Kaufer is now conducting experiments to determine how stress in infancy affects the brain's white matter, and whether chronic early-life stress decreases resilience later in life. She also is looking at the effects of therapies, ranging from exercise to antidepressant drugs, that reduce the impact of stress and stress hormones. It will be interesting to follow her research in this are of brain fitness.

Kaufer believes that moderate or 'good stress'—such as studying hard for an exam or training to compete in the Olympic Games—can build stronger circuitry and a more resilient brain. But acute, prolonged chronic stress wreaks havoc.

We now know the structure of your brain is constantly undergoing changes through plasticity. Mindset, behavior, and chronic stress are never fixed. The power of neuroplasticity makes it possible to change brain structure and function throughout your lifespan. You can consciously make daily lifestyle choices of mindset and behavior that will improve the structure and connectivity of your brain. That's why most of the concentration in this book has been on exposing you to ways to restore your body to balance in order to reduce stress.

5 Simple Strategies to Lower Stress

Best Stress Busters

1. Regular dose of the E-Pill / Physical Activity:

Kick boxing, banging on drums, sparring, pounding the pavement with your sneakers or a punching bag with your fists are terrific ways to recreate the *"fight"* response by letting out aggression (without hurting anyone) and to reduce cortisol.

Any aerobic activity, like walking, jogging, swimming, biking, riding the elliptical... are great ways to recreate the *'flight'* outlet and burn-up cortisol. A little bit of cardio goes a long way. Just 20-30 minutes of activity most days of the week pays huge dividends by lowering cortisol every day and in the long-run.

Fear increases cortisol. Regular physical activity will decrease fear by increasing your self-confidence, resilience, and fortitude—which will reduce cortisol. Yoga will have similar benefits with added benefits of mindfulness training. See the chapter provided in this guide on different types of yoga to try.

If your schedule is too hectic to squeeze in a continuous session of aerobic activity, you can reap the same benefits by breaking daily activity into smaller doses. High intensity Smart Moves circuits like I provide in my resource section are a great place to start. An easy way to guarantee regular activity is to build in intentional lifestyle activity into your daily routine. Try things such as riding a bike to work, walking to the store, taking the stairs instead of the escalator. These all add up to a cumulative tally of reduced cortisol at the end of the day.

2. Mindfulness and Meditation:

Any type of meditation will reduce anxiety and lower cortisol levels. Simply taking a few deep breaths engages the vagus nerve which triggers a signal within your nervous system to slow heart rate, lower blood pressure and decreases cortisol. The next time you feel yourself in a stressful situation that activates your 'Fight-or-Flight' response take 10 deep breaths and feel your entire body relax and decompress.

Setting aside 10-15 minutes to practice mindfulness or meditation will fortify a sense of calm throughout your nervous system, mind, and brain. There are many different types of meditation. "Meditating" doesn't have to be a sacred or a religious experience. People often ask me specifically what kind of meditation I do and how to practice it. I am not an expert on this, but have developed a technique that works for me. I suggest that you do more research, visit a meditation center if you can, and fine-tune a daily meditation practice that fits your schedule and personality. Below is my daily 'meditation routine' and mental practice:

I like to practice this meditation in one 15-minute session. Personally, I like to use a timer and some relaxing music I have on my iTunes. To begin, I usually think of a few words I want to repeat, often I use "One" "Body" "Health". Next, I set my iPad to a 15-minute countdown that ends in a "soft" sound. Then, I sit upright in a chair or sometimes on the floor with my legs crossed at the ankles, set the timer, start the music track and sit with my palms open and fingers interlaced and facing upwards on my knees.

I begin with a "Mindfulness" meditation of simply focusing on my breath and repeating my 'mantra' which is three words that resonate with me (choose your own). You can choose any word or combination of words that have meaning and significance to you. I repeat these words silently in my mind like a rosary as I take deep breaths, relax my shoulders and feel myself drift into a trance-like state.

After a few minutes, I move into the visualization phase I created for restoring balance to my body. I go through a slow deliberate process of seeing oxygen flowing into each organ in my body, delivering nutrients with every inhalation and removing toxins with each exhalation. I used this initially to try best to heal my brain after my stroke, I would visualize blood flowing into the damaged areas of my brain. You may think this is odd, and perhaps it is, but I find it still works for me, and I get to review my anatomy at the same time as I have started to expand my visualization to other parts of the body!

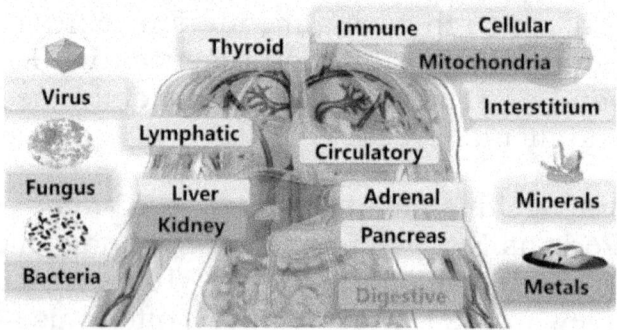

After I've completed this "body systems" cycle, I return back to a single-focused meditation of emptying my mind and focus on my breathing until the soft alarm goes off. When I hear that sound there is always a Pavlovian conditioned response of an 'ahhh' feeling accompanied by a big exhale as I open my eyes and face the real world again.

Remember, you can meditate anytime and any place. There don't have to be strict boundaries to when and how you do it. Mindfulness and meditation is a powerful de-stressor and cortisol reducer that is always in your toolbox and at your fingertips. You can squeeze in a few minutes of meditation on the subway, in a waiting room, on a coffee break... I hope this advice is helpful to you.

3. Social Belonging or Connectivity:

Two studies published recently in the journal *Science* illustrate that social aggression and isolation lead to increased levels of cortisol that trigger a cascade of potential mental health problems, especially in adolescence.

Close knit human bonds, whether it be family, friendship or a romantic partner are vital for your physical and mental health at any age. Recent studies have shown that the vagus nerve also responds to human connectivity and physical touch to relax your parasympathetic nervous system. Perhaps that's why a massage makes you always feel SO good!

The "tend-and-befriend" response is the exact opposite to "fight-or-flight". The "tend-and-befriend" response increases oxytocin and reduces cortisol. Make an effort to spend real face-to-face time with loved ones whenever you can, but even phone calls or Facebook posts can reduce cortisol if they foster a feeling of genuine connectivity.

4. Smiling Laughter and Fun:

Having fun and laughing reduces cortisol levels. Dr. William Fry is an American psychiatrist who has been studying the benefits of laughter for the past 30 years and has found links to laughter and lowered levels of stress hormones. Many studies have shown the benefits of having a sense of humor, laughter and levity. Try to find ways in your daily life to laugh and joke as much as possible and you'll lower cortisol levels.

5. Music and Mood:

Listening to music that you love, and fits whatever mood you're in, has been shown to lower cortisol levels. Music and mood are inherently linked. Scientists continue to uncover how these influences occur at a neural level. Studies prove that the music we listen to engages a wide range of neurobiological systems that affect our psychology and therefore our health. We all know the power of music to improve mood and reduce stress. Add reducing your cortisol levels as another reason to keep the music playing as a soundtrack of health and happiness in your life. Listen to the song *Happy* for example, by the artist Pharrell Williams, and try to keep a sad or stressed face on, bet you can't do it!

Less Caffeine

We Drink it to help Manage the "Stress of Life"

But Here's How Caffeine Really Does Stress Your Body

Caffeine is the most widely used drug in the world and is consumed by more than 100 million Americans each day. It is a potent stimulant and may be consumed in a multitude of forms. These include: coffee, tea, cola drinks, chocolates, cold remedies, pain relievers and dozens of other over-the-counter drugs. So with all this caffeine being used, why are we more tired than ever before?

Why can't a caffcine "fix" fix the problem of us being overstressed and overtired?

Caffeine is a powerful stimulant to nerve tissues. It affects the higher centers of the brain, producing a wakening effect and a more rapid flow of mental processes. It assists the body in overcoming the sense of fatigue, however, it does not relieve it and it does it at a payback "cost" to our bodies. This false energy boost is essentially throttling your hormones and may also be hindering your health efforts. The reason for this is caffeine acts on our adrenal gland (which you learned about in the chapter on stress) and can wear it down causing changes to hormone and blood sugar levels. What results is out-of-balance hormones and dwindling energy.

Think of your car in idle, and now you get in and throttle or rev the gas pedal all day long, on and off until you run out of fuel. You haven't left the yard yet because you haven't put your car in gear to drive, yet you've expended a lot of energy and raced your engine up and down for hours. You probably wouldn't do that to your engine every day because even the sound of your car racing for a few minutes would make you concerned you were doing your car's engine harm, correct? So, why is it OK to throttle your body with caffeine all day? That sometimes edgy, uneasy feeling you get when you need your next fix are a sign your adrenals aren't working properly and you may want to restore your body's natural balance by slowly eliminating caffeine.

More Facts About Caffeine

- Two cups of coffee will cause an increase in hydrochloric acid (HCL) in the stomach for at least an hour. This is a problem for anyone suffering from an ulcer or over-acidity and other digestion problems.
- Caffeine slows the rate of healing of stomach ulcers.
- One cup of coffee will cause a rise in blood pressure.
- Caffeine decreases the body's ability to handle stress.
- In pregnant women, caffeine will enter the fetal circulation in the same concentrations as the mothers. Some research suggests it may be related to birth defects.
- Withdrawal symptoms tend to discourage people from giving up caffeine.
- Continued use of caffeine may lead to insomnia, nervousness, restlessness and even tremors.
- Caffeine masks fatigue when the body needs to rest.
- Caffeine increases respiration rate, urine output and an increase of fatty acids into the bloodstream.

Buyer Beware / The "Fix" is big business

Food and beverage manufacturers are cashing in our your fatigue and need for the next caffeine fix later in the day. They are cranking out record profits on modern day snake oil "energy in a can" with names like Monster, 5-Hour Energy, Red Bull, Rockstar, Jolt, Revive, to name just a few, but all fighting to solve your energy deficit! The added danger to these beverages are young kids are now using them without knowledge of the warnings especially when mixing with alcohol. Deaths reported through ER visits from heart attack and stroke are on the rise due to this alarming trend.

Do you know? 1.5 billion cans of Red Bull were sold in the US alone in 2004 and from that year forward the US energy drink market has exploded by more than 240%. Sales are soon predicted to reach $20 billion!

More Sleep

Rest-Recovery-Restorative Sleep
Your built in tools to enhance fat loss

I group these together again for the sake of time. In reality there are entire books written on each of these topics as they relate to health. My goal here is to point out how the stress cycle needs to be tamed through proper rest or else your health and your waistline will suffer!

Whether it be stress from our jobs, finances, family, or the stress on our bodies from exercise. Doesn't matter what the cause-the stress mechanism is the same. Regardless, when our fight or flight mechanism kicks in, the adrenal glands pump out stress hormones like cortisol and adrenaline, so we are prepared for the challenge. Once, the crisis passes-for example you ran for the train and made it just as the train was set to leave the station- those stress hormones dissipate. But under constant stress from an intense job or deadline, or constant worries over money or relationships, those same hormones stay high.

Research is showing that elevated levels of these hormones can make fat loss difficult because cortisol increases hunger and can trigger cravings for starchy foods that provide quick energy. So, it is easy to say don't worry and you'll lose weight but in reality it is not that simple.

Solving your stress problems is certainly not in the scope of my expertise, but I wanted to point out this factor and connect it to your weight loss efforts so that you may begin to seek help from other professionals or find resources to develop strategies to improve your environment.

Studies show most of us are sleep deprived

In a recent sleep study conducted by the National Sleep Foundation, seventy-four percent of us have trouble sleeping at least two nights a week. Not only does lack of sleep make us tired, grumpy and angry at the world, new research also is showing that chronic sleep loss may be making us fat.

A recent study conducted of over 8,000 participants in Japan found that those who slept less than 8 hours a night were three times as likely to be obese than those who normally sleep 10 hours or more.

The reason being studied is that much like the response demonstrated above to stress, fatigue is a stressor and a tired body tends to elevate cortisol levels to compensate. How can this lower metabolism? It is now theorized that these elevated cortisol levels can reduce glucose tolerance and thyroid hormone levels, which may contribute to insulin resistance and a sluggish metabolism.

Sleep and rest (power naps too) are important to restoring physiological balance- it gives your body time out of that stress/feedback loop that I described earlier earlier in the section on strategies to reduce stress. When your body does not have down time to recover, it ultimately goes into a primitive protective mode, and begins to store calories as fat rather than use them for energy. Protect your health and recharge your batteries, make time for sleep!

David Dansereau

References and Resources on Obesity
More Obesity Stats and References

AMERICA'S OBESITY EPIDEMIC
Today, two thirds of adults and nearly one in three children struggle with overweight and obesity. Twenty years ago, no state had an obesity rate above 15 percent. Today, more than two out of three states, 38 total, have obesity rates over 25 percent, according to Trust for America's Health. The rate of childhood obesity more than doubled from 1980 to 2000; 30 states have child obesity rates of 30 percent or more.

OBESITY'S IMPACT ON AMERICA'S HEALTH
Obesity is linked to more than 60 chronic diseases. According to the American Cancer Society, obese adults are at increased risk for all cancers.
Obesity contributes to two-thirds of all heart disease, according to the CDC.
66 percent of American adults with doctor-diagnosed arthritis are overweight or obese.
Over 75 percent of hypertension cases are directly related to obesity.
More than 80 percent of people with type 2 diabetes are overweight.

THE ECONOMIC IMPACT OF OBESITY

In 2010, the nonpartisan Congressional Budget Office reported that nearly 20 percent of the increase in U.S. health care spending (from 1987-2007) was caused by obesity. The annual health costs related to obesity in the U.S. are as high as $168 billion, and nearly 17 percent of U.S. medical costs can be attributed on obesity, according to research released by the National Bureau of Economic Research.

OBESITY'S IMPACT ON THE WORKFORCE
Full-time workers in the U.S. who are overweight or obese and have other chronic health conditions miss an estimated 450 million additional days of work each year compared with healthy workers — resulting in an estimated cost of more than $153 billion in lost productivity annually, according to a 2011 Gallup Poll.

Medical expenses for obese employees are 42 percent higher than for a person with a healthy weight, according to the Centers for Disease Control.

OBESITY'S IMPACT ON COMMUNITIES OF NEED
Blacks, Hispanics and Native people are much more likely to be obese than whites, according to CDC data.

Low-income neighborhoods are more affected by obesity than affluent areas, reflecting a range of policy and cultural influences.

OBESITY AND PHYSICAL ACTIVITY
Approximately 50 percent of children walked or bicycled to school in 1969; today, fewer than 15 percent of schoolchildren walk or bike to school, according to the Safe Routes to School Partnership.

Only 3.8 percent of U.S. elementary schools, 7.9 percent of U.S. middle schools and 2.1 percent of U.S. high schools provide daily physical education for students, according to the Centers for Disease Control.

52 percent of adults do not meet <u>minimum</u> physical activity recommendations.

OBESITY AND NUTRITION

Only 12 percent of adults and two percent of children eat a healthy diet consistent with federal nutrition recommendations.

According to the USDA, healthier diets could prevent at least $71 billion per year in medical costs, lost productivity and lost lives.

1. CDC: "The Association Between School-Based Physical Activity, Including Physical Education, and Academic Performance"
2. CDC: "Physical Activity and the Health of Young People"
3. Duke Global Health Institute: "Obese Workers Cost Workplace More Than Medical Expenses, Absenteeism"
4. Gallup: "The Cost of Obesity to U.S. Cities
5. McKinsey Quarterly: "The real cost of obesity"
6. National Bureau of Economic Research: "The Medical Care Costs of Obesity: An Instrumental Variables Approach "Thomson Reuters: "Obesity in the Workforce: Health Effects and Healthcare Costs"

Summary: Weight Loss Guidelines

Here's the latest American College of Cardiology / American Heart /Stroke Association Weight Loss Guidelines

New ACC/AHA Prevention Guidelines were developed in 2013 to address blood cholesterol, obesity, healthy living and risk assessment. The following are 10 points to remember about these American College of Cardiology (ACC)/American Heart Association (AHA)/The Obesity Society (TOS) Guideline on the best advice for Management of Overweight and Obesity in Adults. These recommendations are based on the latest scientific evidence from 133 research studies. This data represents the most current studies that has been conducted since the release of the last guidelines 15 years ago.

The expert panel that wrote the report was convened by the Unites States National Heart, Lung, and Blood Institute (NHLBI) of the National Institutes of Health. At the invitation of the NHLBI, the American Heart Association, the American College of Cardiology and The Obesity Society officially assumed the joint governance, management and publication of these obesity guidelines in June 2013. Committee members volunteered their time and were required to disclose all healthcare-related relationships, including those existing one year before the initiation of the writing project. What follows is my summary of the top ten key points related to these guidelines.

David Dansereau

Summary of the Top 10 Points - Obesity Guidelines

1. Approximately 78 million adults in the United States are obese, which places them at risk for morbidity from a variety of conditions including diabetes, coronary heart disease, and stroke. An expert panel was assembled to first develop a list of critical questions to be addressed. Five targeted questions were selected based on relevance to health care providers who frequently work with obese patients, and to provide an update on the benefits and risks of weight loss achieved with various approaches. Not included were questions related to genetics of obesity, binge eating disorders, pharmacotherapy, and cost-effectiveness of interventions to manage obesity. Five critical questions were addressed, which centered around evidence for:

Weight loss and reduction of cardiovascular disease (CVD) risk factors, events, and mortality;

Current cut points for body mass index (BMI) and waist circumference in relation to CVD risk;

Different diets in relation to weight loss and weight maintenance;

Comprehensive lifestyle intervention programs for weight loss and maintenance of weight loss; and

Bariatric surgery for weight loss, and maintenance of weight loss, and impact on CVD risk factors and mortality over the short- and long-term.

2. Providers are recommended to measure height and weight and calculate BMI at annual visits or more frequently to identify patients who need to lose weight. Use of current cut points for overweight (BMI >25.0-29.9

kg/m2) and obesity (BMI ≥30 kg/m2) should be continued to identify adults who may be at increased risk for CVD. A cut point for obesity (BMI ≥30 kg/m2) should be used to identify adults at increased risk for all-cause mortality. Patients who are overweight or obese should be counseled that their BMI level places them at increased risk for CVD, type 2 diabetes, and all-cause mortality.

3. Waist circumference should be measured at annual visits or more frequently in overweight and obese adults. Cut points for increased waist circumference defined by the National Institutes of Health or World Health Organization (>35 inches or 88 cm for women and >40 inches or 102 cm for men) can be used. Patients who have an increased waist circumference should be counseled that their BMI level places them at increased risk for CVD, type 2 diabetes, and all-cause mortality.

4. Overweight and obese adults with CVD risk factors (including elevated blood pressure, hyperlipidemia, and hyperglycemia) should be counseled that even modest weight loss (3-5% of body weight) can result in clinically meaningful benefits for triglycerides, blood glucose, glycated hemoglobin, and development of diabetes (type 2). Greater weight loss (>5%) can further reduce blood pressure, improve lipids (both low-density lipoprotein and high-density lipoprotein cholesterol), and reduce need of medications to control blood pressure, blood glucose, and lipids.

5. A diet prescribed for weight loss is recommended to be part of a comprehensive lifestyle intervention, a component of which includes a plan to achieve reduced caloric intake. Any one of the following methods can be used to reduce food and calorie intake:

Prescribe 1,200-1,500 kcal/day for women and 1,500-

1,800 kcal/day for men (kcal levels are usually adjusted for the individual's body weight);

Prescribe a 500 kcal/day or 750 kcal/day energy deficit; or

Prescribe one of the evidence-based diets that restricts certain food types (such as high-carbohydrate foods, low-fiber foods, or high-fat foods) in order to create an energy deficit by reduced food intake.

6. Prescribing a calorie-restricted diet should be based on the patient's preferences, health status, and preferably with a referral to a nutrition professional for counseling.

7. Overweight and obese adults who would benefit from weight loss are recommended to participate in at least 6 months of a comprehensive lifestyle program, which assists participants to adhere to a lower calorie diet and to increase physical activity. Such programs are recommended to include high-intensity (i.e., ≥14 sessions in 6 months), comprehensive weight loss interventions provided in individual or group sessions by a trained interventionist. Electronically delivered weight loss programs (including by telephone) that include personalized feedback from a trained interventionist can be prescribed for weight loss, but may result in smaller weight loss than face-to-face interventions. Some commercial-based programs that provide a comprehensive lifestyle intervention can be prescribed as an option for weight loss, provided there is peer-reviewed published evidence of their safety and efficacy.

8. It is recommended that very low-calorie diets (defined as <800 kcal/day) be used only when medical monitoring and trained providers are available, and only as part of a high-intensity lifestyle intervention.

9. Weight loss maintenance is recommended to be a component of patients' overall weight loss plan. Participation in a long-term (≥1 year) comprehensive weight loss maintenance program is strongly recommended. Programs should include regular contact with trained personnel, face-to-face or telephone-delivered, to encourage high levels of physical activity (200-300 minutes/week), monitor body weight (at least weekly), and adhere to a reduced-calorie diet (needed to maintain lower body weight).

10. Among adults with a BMI ≥40 or BMI ≥35 with obesity-related comorbid conditions, who have not responded to behavioral treatments with or without pharmacotherapy, bariatric surgery may be an appropriate option. For individuals with a BMI <35, there is insufficient evidence to recommend for or against undergoing bariatric surgical procedures.

The link to the full report, "2013 ACC/AHA Guideline for the Management of Overweight and Obesity in Adults" is available in the Resources Chapter.

Weight Management University

On-line Resource Replaces Weight-Loss Marketing Hype with Real World Science-Based Education

-Press Release-

Attleboro, MA [Jan 1, 2014] – **PTC Physical Therapy Consulting** – a leader in professional health education, fitness and lifestyle, announced today the launch of its Weight-Management University-101 (WMU-101). It is a self-paced, 12-session curriculum that covers a range of topics from – "how your body processes food" to "how your body burns fat." In direct contrast to quick-fix diet programs, Weight-Management University-101 is the "adult conversation" regarding both weight and overall health management.

The WMU-101 program provides an online, multi-media education teaching the basics of human physiology in a fun, interactive and easy-to-understand format using "lay terms" throughout several mediums including:

- high-definition videos audio downloads (.mp3 files)
- document downloads (.pdf files)
- multiple choice quizzes

The course is specifically designed to help people understand the real physiology behind long-term weight-management – with a focus on exercise and body-composition rather than pounds-on-the-scale as a metric. "Education is the key to empowerment and success," says David Dansereau, MSPT, Owner and Founder of PTC Physical Therapy Consulting and Weight Management University. "So, the very first step to long-term weight-management is to understand how the human body actually functions.

> *"WMU-101 is the perfect tool for our one on one clinic, virtual online clients, as well as for schools and our corporate wellness participants to learn the science and physiology behind managing their weight, increasing energy, handling stress and creating their own feelings of health and well-being."-DP Dansereau,MSPT*

Even after the comprehensive 12-session curriculum is completed, our clients can still access WMU-101 and use it as a "knowledge resource" in order to review the materials regarding long-term weight-management, nutrition or wellness protocol.

The online content and high-definition videos display on all digital platforms from mobile phones, tablets and laptops to desktops and large screen projectors. This allows participants to access WMU-101 from home, work or anywhere internet access is available.

Learn more at wmu-101.com

David Dansereau

Bright Minds Kids Campaign

Why Nutrition Education is Needed Now in Schools and Communities

Here's the Facts: "Only 12 percent of adults and two percent of children currently eat a healthy diet. Only 3.8 percent of U.S. elementary schools, 7.9 percent of U.S. middle schools and 2.1 percent of U.S. high schools provide daily physical education for students, according to the Centers for Disease Control".

> **"Something has to change dramatically in our school and medical / health education system as clearly our young <u>Bright Minds</u> are not receiving adequate exercise and nutrition education to help protect their health."**
>
> -David Dansereau,MSPT PTC Physical Therapy

Growing Nutrition "Debt"

Sadly we continue graduating kids that know little about good nutrition and positive exercise behaviors. Not knowing about how your body works puts kids at higher risk of a nutrition "debt" that we all pay back later in the form of a host of known health complications associated with obesity and increased medical costs. One of my goals in offering this course is to give every classroom that would like access to this peer reviewed nutrition and exercise content the ability to quickly implement a cost effective nutrition and healthy lifestyle curriculum. Ask us about our WMU classroom packs and corporate sponsor matching course enrollment opportunities, we need beta testers to create a "**WIN/WIN**" Community

Nutrition Education learning partnership where we match corporations with struggling schools. Together with WMU we can get your community out of "nutrition" debt!

Kids need a "University Quality" Nutrition Education to learn how their bodies work well BEFORE they actually get to college!

-DP Dansereau PTC Physical Therapy

Want to Join our Educated Nutrition Community and offer WMU Diplomas to your Classroom or Group?

The release of WMU-101 provides an affordable opportunity to bring an engaging nutrition and healthy lifestyle exercise intervention into your medical facility, school or organization, without the "heavy lifting" and expenses involved with marketing, ordering textbooks, preparing lesson plans or hiring a new wellness staff.

A portion of all book proceeds from Body in Balance go to support my Bright Minds Campaign. Visit my partners page at wmu-101.com

David Dansereau

More Online Resources for this Book

Resources

Please visit my resource page for products and materials mentioned in this guide. Check back often as I'll be loading in more information and announcing free webinars to help you get your Body in Balance.

Visit www.smartmovesguidebook.com

GMO Nation

The naked truth about the genetic engineering experiment that is on your plate and what it means to your body.

Here's why:
The genetically modified foods controversy currently brewing in the US and worldwide is a dispute over the use of food and other goods derived from genetically modified crops instead of from conventional crops, and other uses of genetic engineering in food production. The dispute involves consumers, biotechnology companies, governmental regulators, non-governmental organizations, scientists and universities that are in many cases funded to promote biotech. The key areas of controversy related to genetically modified food are: whether GM food should be labeled, the role of government regulators, the effect of GM crops on health and the environment, the effect on pesticide resistance, the impact of GM crops for farmers, and the role of GM crops in feeding the world population. All these issues are being wrestled with throughout the world as well and genetic engineering and food security controversies which cut to the core of just who has the right to mess with Mother Nature. The big agricultural giants like Monsanto and Dow chemical are working hard to do just that by manipulating GM seeds with little concern for human and environmental safety. What I have included in this chapter is more background on GMOs so you can make an educated decision on your own.

Where are GMOs and how did they get into our food?

GMOs were first introduced into the food supply in the mid-1990s, GMOs are now present in the vast majority of processed foods in the US. While they are banned as food ingredients in Europe and elsewhere, the FDA does not even require the labeling of GMOs in food ingredient lists.

Although there have been attempts to increase nutritional benefits or productivity, the two main traits that have been added to date are herbicide tolerance and the ability of the plant to produce its own pesticide. These results have no health benefit, only economic benefit.

What foods are GM?

Currently commercialized GM crops in the U.S. include soy (94%), cotton (90%), canola (90%), sugar beets (95%), corn (88%), Hawaiian papaya (more than 50%), zucchini and yellow squash (over 24,000 acres).

Products derived from the above, including oils from all four, soy protein, soy lecithin, cornstarch, corn syrup and high fructose corn syrup among others. There are also many "invisible ingredients," derived from GM crops that are not obviously from corn or soy. Be aware that GMO ingredients have other names and they may be difficult to spot.

Some hidden GMO ingredients include: aspartame, baking soda, caramel color, corn flour, corn sugar, corn syrup, dextrose, fructose, protein, lecithin, malt, maltodextrin, sorbitol, sugar, soy sauce, soy lecithin, vitamin E, vitamin B12, and xanthum gum. Check your food labels and you'll quickly discover when you match up these ingredients on the list you have indeed been unknowingly filling your shopping cart and serving up your families hefty portions of GMOs for years, especially if you purchase prepackaged convenience foods or dine out frequently.

Why should you care?

Genetically modified foods have been linked to toxic and allergic reactions, sick, sterile, and dead livestock, and damage to virtually every organ studied in lab animals. The effects on humans of consuming these new combinations of proteins produced in GMOs are unknown and have not been studied. So how can they be assumed safe to eat?

GMO Health Effects Ignored in the US

The American Academy of Environmental Medicine (AAEM) doesn't think GMOs are safe. The Academy reported that "Several animal studies indicate serious health risks associated with GM food," including infertility, immune problems, accelerated aging, faulty insulin regulation, and changes in major organs and the gastrointestinal system. The AAEM asked physicians to advise patients to avoid GM foods.

Before the FDA decided to allow GMOs into food without labeling, FDA scientists had repeatedly warned that GM foods can create unpredictable, hard-to-detect side effects, including allergies, toxins, new diseases, and nutritional problems. They urged long-term safety studies, but were ignored because of inside connections that the FDA has with big-agricultural giants like Monsanto. In the US, these failed Federal policies and special deals are allowing politics and not science to set the agenda for our GMO Nation.

Since then, findings include:

- Thousands of sheep, buffalo, and goats in India died after grazing on Bt cotton plants
- Mice eating GM corn for the long term had fewer, and smaller, babies

- More than half the babies of mother rats fed GM soy died within three weeks, and were smaller
- Testicle cells of mice and rats on GM soy change significantly
- By the third generation, most GM soy-fed hamsters lost the ability to have babies
- Rodents fed GM corn and soy showed immune system responses and signs of toxicity
- Cooked GM soy contains as much as 7-times the amount of a known soy allergen
- Soy allergies skyrocketed by 50% in the UK, soon after GM soy was introduced
- The stomach lining of rats fed GM potatoes showed excessive cell growth, a condition that may lead to cancer.
- Studies showed organ lesions, altered liver and pancreas cells, changed enzyme levels, etc.

Unlike safety evaluations for drugs, there are no human clinical trials of GM foods

The only published human feeding experiment revealed that the genetic material inserted into GM soy transfers into bacteria living inside our intestines and continues to function. This means that long after we stop eating GM foods, we may still have their GM proteins produced continuously inside us. This could mean:

- If the antibiotic gene inserted into most GM crops were to transfer, it could create super diseases, resistant to antibiotics
- If the gene that creates Bt-toxin in GM corn were to transfer, it might turn our intestinal bacteria into living pesticide factories.

Although no studies have evaluated if antibiotic or Bt-toxin genes transfer, that is one of the key problems. The safety assessments are too superficial to even identify most of the potential dangers from GMOs.

Recent health studies throughout the world provide growing evidence of harm from GMOs:

> "GM Corn Damages Liver and Kidneys"-*truth-out.org*
> "Meat Raised on GM Feed is Different"-*comcom.govt.nz*
> "Roundup Could Cause Birth Defects"-*laht.com*
> "Genetically Modified Soy Linked to Sterility"-*responsibletechnology.org*

What Does the Rest of the World Think About GMO's?

Today, over 50 countries around the globe including Australia, Japan and all of the countries in the European Union have restrictions and even bans on the production, and sale of GMOs. Yet in our GMO Nation (US), we keep pumping them on American plates and there are countless other GE varieties in development for just about every fruit and vegetable variety imagined. The United States is currently the largest commercial producer of genetically modified crops on the planet.

> *"If people let the government decide what foods they eat and what medicines they take, their bodies will soon be in as sorry a state as the souls who live under tyranny."* -Thomas Jefferson

Long Term Effects of GMOs on the Environment

Crops such as Bt cotton produce pesticides inside the plant. This kills or deters insects, saving the farmer from having to spray pesticides. The plants themselves are toxic, and not just to insects. For example, farmers in India, who let their sheep graze on Bt cotton plants after the harvest, saw thousands of sheep die!

Herbicide tolerance lets the farmer spray weed-killer *directly* on the crop without killing it. Comparative studies on the toxic residues in foods from such crops have not yet been done.

Pollen from GM crops can contaminate nearby crops of the same type, except for soy, which does not cross-pollinate. In fact, virtually all heritage varieties of corn in Mexico (the origin of all corn) have been found to have some contamination. Canola and cotton also cross-pollinate. The long-term effects on the environment could be disastrous. Bee populations have been dropping dramatically, and there are most likely more than one area to point the finger at as to the cause, but bee farmers from thoughout the US and Canada have reported entire hive deaths when nearby farms spray with GM herbicides.

Epidemiological studies on the herbicide Roundup developed by multinational Monsanto show links with many serious health problems

> *Research has found that "pure glyphosate, in doses lower than those used in common farm fumigation, causes defects ... (and) could be interfering in some normal embryonic development mechanism having to do with the way in which cells divide and die."*

Epidemiological studies show a link between Roundup /glyphosate exposure and serious health problems, including:

- DNA damage
- Premature births and miscarriages
- Birth defects including neural tube defects and anencephaly (absence of a large part of the brain and skull)
- Multiple myeloma, a type of cancer
- Non-Hodgkin's lymphoma, a type of cancer
- Disruption of neurobehavioral development in children of pesticide applicators – in particular, attention-deficit disorder (ADD) and attention-deficit hyperactivity disorder (ADHD).
- Environmental impact: Glyphosate does not degrade so we do not have a way of measuring long term compounded exposure.

Epidemiological studies cannot prove a cause-and-effect relationship between exposure to a suspect substance and a health effect. However, in the case of glyphosate/Roundup, toxicological studies carried out under controlled laboratory conditions confirm the causal relationship to health problems.

In our GMO Nation people are widely exposed to glyphosate

Glyphosate-based herbicides are widely used outside of the farm environment – for example, by municipal authorities to control weeds on roadsides and in parks and school grounds, as well as by home gardeners who often spray them liberally throughout their lawns and gardens to compound the environmental exposure dose we already receive. So even when farm use is excluded, people's exposure to glyphosate is significant. In agricultural areas where GM glyphosate-resistant crops are grown, it is not uncommon for spraying to go on right next to schools and farms that may not even know they have been exposed! These same crops and seeds that are "Roundup Ready" are then fed to much of the livestock including fish and poultry confined and force fed an unnatural diet of these GMO soy and corn feed.

Published papers telling us that GMO foods "are safe and necessary to sustain world demand for food" are most often authored by scientists that have been hired by biotech companies. Many argue that these same authorities who are speaking in favor of GMO are being fortified through joint ventures, lucrative consultancies and sponsorship of scientific forums in university departments that ultimately compromise the academic science.

[Personal Sidebar] You may already be aware that I support the efforts for GMO Labeling in my home state (Rhode Island). Most of what is in this chapter came from my research I provided for testimony at the Rhode Island State House explaining my position as a health professional on why GMO labeling is needed. You can see a copy of my testimony on the resources links for this book as well an article I wrote about what I uncovered at the University of Rhode Island at their recent GMO Food Safety Conference. Since I testified for GMO labeling, there have been some interesting developments and more concern for GMO and glyphosate usage. I have outlined a few of these significant headlines and developments below.

World Health Organization (WHO) Report on glyphosate and cancer risk

An ingredient in Monsanto's Roundup weed-killer – glyphosate – is "probably carcinogenic," according to a decision and report by the World Health Organization (WHO). The decision was laid out in a recent report in The Lancet Oncology, and is now published on the WHO's

International Agency for Research on Cancer (IARC) website. The analysis is based on the existing research on the chemical exposure in people and lab animals. What does it mean? If nothing else, at least the new decision by the WHO will raise awareness on the part of the customer – and hopefully the concerns and fears it may also spark will turn into energies in the right direction: A demand for greater food safety and more scientific studies on the effects of these chemicals have on us and the environment in the long-run.

New England Journal of Medicine Article Calls for FDA to Require Mandatory Labeling of FDA Foods

Monsanto and the fast food industry like to say that people who want GMOs to be labeled are anti-science. But after an important article appeared on August 20th, they'll have an awfully hard time calling the New England Journal of Medicine anti-science. In this recent issue of the New England Journal of Medicine, two respected experts on pesticides and children's environmental health call for the FDA to require mandatory labeling of GMO foods.

What the article says:

In the article, titled "<u>GMOs, Herbicides, and Public Health</u>," Dr. Philip J. Landrigan, the Dean for Global Health at Mount Sinai School of Medicine, and co-author Charles Benbrook, a crop and soil scientist, say the time has come for three important steps. One of these is GMO labeling. They write:

"We believe the time has come to revisit the United States' reluctance to label GM foods."

As they explain, two recent developments are dramatically changing the GMO landscape: The number of chemical herbicides applied to GM crops has increased sharply and is scheduled to increase even more in the next few years. This year, the International Agency for Research on Cancer classified glyphosate, the herbicide used most widely on GM crops, as a "probable human carcinogen." And the agency classified 2,4-D, another herbicide, as a "possible human carcinogen."

The authors believe labeling will have multiple benefits. It will help track the emergence of new food allergies and better evaluate the effects of chemical herbicides applied to GM foods. And also, it will respect the wishes of the growing numbers of consumers who insist they have a right to know what is in the foods and beverages they are buying.

The article also calls for the National Toxicology Program to urgently assess the nature, effects, and possible poisons in pure glyphosate, formulated glyphosate, and mixtures of glyphosate and other herbicides.
Finally, the article calls for the EPA to delay its implementation of its decision to allow the use of Enlist Duo, a combination herbicide made with both glyphosate and 2,4-D that is designed for use on GMO crops.
The authors say the data supporting the herbicide combination is flawed and doesn't consider more recent studies showing the potential health effects in infants and children.

U.S. Right to Know -INVESTIGATION OF BIG FOOD AND ITS FRONT GROUPS

U.S. Right to Know (usrtk.org) is a new nonprofit food organization that investigates and reports on what food companies don't want us to know about our food. At the time of this writing they were conducting an ongoing investigation into the collusion between Big Food, its front groups, and university faculty and staff to deliver industry PR to the public. Thus far, they have reported "it has been fruitful", and their work was reported on in a New York Times Report on Sept 5, 2015 entitled:

"*Food Industry Enlisted Academics in G.M.O. Lobbying War, Emails Show*" –New York Times

The Times article links emails obtained via state Freedom of Information Act requests filed by U.S. Right to Know. These emails reveal how Monsanto and its partners use so-called "independent" third-party scientists and professors to deliver their PR messaging. Since the companies themselves are not credible messengers, they use these scientists and professors as shills to shape the media narrative on food issues, particularly GMOs.

According to the U.S. Right to Know website and report this is a key part of Big Food's PR strategy. "The agrichemical and food industries are spending vast sums* of money to convince the public that their food, crops, GMOs, additives and pesticides are safe, desirable and healthy. "

*(Since 2012, the agrichemical and food industries have mounted a complex, multifaceted public relations, advertising, lobbying and political campaign in the United States, costing more than $100 milion, to defend genetically engineered food and crops and the pesticides that accompany them.)

U.S. Right to Know has filed state Freedom of Information Acts requests to try to obtain the emails and documents of 43 public university faculty and staff, to learn more about this public relations effort. Thus far, they have reported having received documents in nine of these requests.

U.S. Right to Know cites they have requested records from scientists, economists, law professors, extension specialists and communicators. All work in public institutions, funded by the taxpayers. They believe the public deserves to know more about the flow of money and level of coordination between public university scientists and other academics, and the agrichemical and food companies whose interests they promote.

At this point, there is no evidence that academic work was compromised, but the emails show how academics have shifted from researchers to actors in lobbying and corporate public relations campaigns.

One thing is Clear, there are many BIG players in the Food Safety Debate

Even with all the new momentum by food advocacy groups and the anger expressed through public opinion polls in the U.S. and around the world, there is a looming momentum killer in the U.S. that will further anger public concerns and be a real killer for food policy progress. Currently, the FDA does not require labeling of genetically modified foods, even though 65 countries mandate the labeling of GM foods, and more than 90 percent of Americans support it. Perhaps knowing the issue of GM food safety is such a growing public health concern, our political leaders have either steered clear of taking a position, used it to gain votes, or have been influenced by lobbyists to remain loyal to big food industry and their profits over prevention of public harm.

Consider this- In 2007, as a presidential candidate, then-Senator Obama promised mandatory labeling of genetically engineered foods. He said: "Here's what I'll do as president ... We'll let folks know if their food has been genetically modified, because Americans should know what they're buying," Obama has yet to keep his promise and in fact is now in favor of new "anti-right to know" food policy legislation.

The Potential Non GMO / Clean Food Momentum Killer

Recently, The Safe and Accurate Food Labeling Act of 2015 (or the DARK Act-a nickname given by its opponents-"Deny Americans the Right to Know"), which would block states and federal government from making mandatory labeling laws, passed in the House. At this writing, it was waiting to go to vote in the Senate. This proposal is also being referred to by opponents as the "Monsanto Protection Act" because it would prohibit individual state's right to label GMO foods.

Bottom Line: What is Big Food hiding from?

If they were indeed providing such a great product and were engaged in true public policy and community health concerns, why these mega food giants need to lobby the government for protection and also want in some cases to change their name?

According to U.S. Right to Know non-profit, Monsanto propose resently to change its name to escape negative PR woes. "In a 2014 Harris Poll gauging the reputations of major corporations, Monsanto's "reputation quotient" ranked 58 out of 60 companies. In other words, it was the third most hated company measured." When this is all said and done I think we will find a real smoking gun here (similar to big tobacco cover up) as to what is keeping many bodies out of balance and sick. The naked truth is the answer may now be on our plates. What are the long term consequences of these hormone disrupting chemicals, new GMO foods and foreign food allergens we are now exposed to daily doing to our health? Furthermore, why are we (U.S.) about to allow even more inadequately tested genetically modified foods / herbicide resistant crops into the marketplace? Many, many more GM foods are in the pipeline and currently being developed. Mother nature has a way to try to restore balance, but in this case, she could be overwhelmed and in the end this unregulated food experiment could prove lethal. I indeed hope I am wrong in my observations, but from all I have studied, I strongly do believe we are presently going down the wrong food path.

Take Action: Get started saying "No" to GMO

To eliminate GMO's now, begin to shop organic and look for the "non-gmo label or non-gmo verified" statement and logo on packaged items. In the references link I provide a great shopping app and tipsheet to help you.

What if I buy only "Natural" products? They must be non-GMO, right?

Wrong. The "Natural" label is a sham.

Consumer Reports tested several products that are labeled as "Natural" because they found that the majority of Americans still believe that the "Natural" label means that they are non-GMO. As I've written about in the past on my nutrition website (my-nutrition-coach.com), the word "Natural" on a product means absolutely nothing in regards to GMOs - the FDA has failed to define the use of this term which allows food manufacturers to deceptively label their products as "Natural" to trick us into thinking their product is better than the others on the shelf. Consumer Reports notes that, *"Consumers who want to avoid GE ingredients should not rely on products labeled "natural" to avoid GMOs. This label is highly confusing and generally misleading for consumers and Consumer Reports is asking the government to ban its use on food"*. They should - because GMOs are not natural.

Yet, GMOs remain in "Natural" foods all over the country.

David Dansereau

Consumer Reports found that some "Natural" products contained similar amounts of GMOs as their counterparts without a natural label. For instance, they found substantial quantities of GMO corn or GMO soy in popular "Natural" foods such as Kashi GoLean Honey & Cinnamon hot cereal (owned by Kellogg's), Utz All Natural Multigrain Tortillas, and Nature Valley Crunchy Oats 'N Honey Granola Bars (owned by General Mills). Here's the full list from Consumer Reports:

Products guilty of using GMOs (A-Z):

Betty Crocker Authentic Cornbread & Muffin Mix
Boca Original Vegan Veggie Burgers
Corn Tortillas/Tortilla Flour
Doritos Oven Baked Nacho Cheese
Enfamil ProSobee Soy Infant Formula
General Mills Cocoa Puffs
General Mills Corn Chex
General Mills Kix
General Mills Trix
Gerber Good Start Soy
Jiffy Corn Muffin Mix
Kashi GoLean (in the process of of getting Non-GMO project verified)
Kashi GoLean Hearty Honey & Cinnamon (Hot Cereal)
Kellogg's Froot Loops
Kellogg's Special K Protein Chocolatey Peanut Butter Granola Snack Bar
Krusteaz Natural Honey Cornbread & Muffin Mix
La Banderita Corn Tortillas
Maseca Instant Corn Masa Flour
Mission White Corn Tortillas
Mission Yellow Corn Tortillas
MorningStar Farms Chik'n Nuggets
MorningStar Farms Grillers California Turk'y Burger
Nature Valley Crunchy Oats 'N Honey Granola Bars

Nature Valley Protein Peanut Butter Dark Chocolate Chewy Bar
Nice! Oats & Honey Crunchy Granola Bar (Walgreens)
Old El Paso Crunchy Taco Shells
Ortega Yellow Corn Taco Shells
PowerBar Performance Energy Chocolate Peanut Butter
Quaker Life Original
Quaker Yellow Corn Meal
Similac Go & Grow Soy Infant Formula
Similac Soy Isomil
Snyder's of Hanover Yellow Corn Tortilla Chips
Tostitos Multigrain Tortilla Chips

Wrap Up-What Does this Naked Truth Mean

To Get a Body Back in Balance

It is Simple. One of the take away lessons I hope you keep from this book is that you certainly can change many of your nutrition and exercise habits almost instantly. It is often more important to know what to eliminate, and why, than to worry about what to eat. That's why this is not a "diet" book. You have ultimate power with your fork. You and I may never be able to change food policies at state and federal levels because lobbyists will always fight for the good of profit over prevention. But now you are informed and can do more reading on these topics if they struck a nerve with you too. It is important to know you can and should still try to eat clean, and you will have an impact by not purchasing those unhealthy foods for you and your family. Simple tweaks are able to disrupt the food system in a positive way, and proper knowledge of how and why your body responds to the right dosage of each of these health elements can be passed down to our young bright minds to promote a healthier generation.

You CAN succeed. You CAN be healthy again and you can feed your DNA to get well and move to pump vital healing oxygen to your cells to restore balance. But it can never happen as long as you're holding on to excuses. Many times we get caught up in all the obstacles we're up against that others aren't, and many times, those excuses cause us to delay taking action toward becoming better (and healthier).

"If only [fill in the excuse here] , then I'd get started."

No, get started today!! If you are reading this, it means you have completed the this book and you now have the "skillpower" to achieve your goals.

You see, there's a 100% chance you won't achieve your goals if you don't get started. And every day that goes by where that start is delayed, is another day that you accept living a life less than your best.

That's no way to live, and you deserve better than that. You deserve your best. You deserve living, breathing, and enjoying each day at its full potential.

But how can you achieve that?

Avoid the biggest health sabotaging "danger zone"- Drop the excuses and get started today.

It doesn't matter if everyone in your family is overweight. You can be thin.

It doesn't matter if you are currently in pain and taking multiple medications. You can restore mobility, have more energy and move pain free again.

It doesn't matter if your schedule is jammed packed from morning until night. You can prioritize and find time for your health through choosing proper nutrition and productive exercise. It doesn't matter how much money you make. There are many "cheap", healthy options available.

But in order to SEE the solutions, you first have to let go of all the reasons why you can't...because reality is, you CAN.

So, one last reminder...you can't change your genetics, but you can change your attitude, your persistence, your environment and what you expose your body to, the people you listen to and hang around with, and the things you do. So in these ways, when you move and take action you can influence your DNA so if you want to, just get started.

You can be great. You can soar. You can achieve a healthier you and you must do so because your health is your most valuable asset and you should be protecting it daily with nourishing foods and therapeutic exercise.

"Where there is a will, there's a way". It's cliche, but it couldn't be more true. That was one of my father's favorite lines and as a kid it drove me nuts every time I was frustrated and I found my dad reciting this line to me to keep trying. Guess what, it stuck and I am passing that cliche on to you! He also would back that line up with another of his favorite one-liners- *"You quit, you lose"* if he felt I needed another reminder of what would happen if I gave up. So, don't quit, you now have the skillpower to make change happen.

When you want it, there's nothing that can hold you back...no obstacle too big...no excuse worth giving the time of day. Just get started today. Make the commitment...not another day goes by leaning on excuses, starting right now. You're BETTER than that and I know you want it or you wouldn't have reached the end of this book.

Start now! You can do it!!

I wish you all the best on your own health journey,

David

Body in Balance

Get the Latest Books in the Smart Moves Guidebook Series

www.ingramcontent.com/pod-product-compliance
Lightning Source LLC
Chambersburg PA
CBHW051631170526
45167CB00001B/143